The Healing Power of Soy

The Enlightened Person's Guide to Nature's Wonder Food

D1373031

Carol Ann Rinzler

PRIMA HEALTH
A Division of Prima Publishing

PRIMA HEALTH and colophon are trademarks of Prima Communications, Inc.

Warning—Disclaimer
This book is not intended to provide medical advice and is sold with the understanding that the publisher and the author are not liable for the misconception or misuse of information provided. The author and Prima Publishing shall have neither liability nor responsibility to any person or entity with respect to any loss, damage, or injury caused or alleged to be caused directly or indirectly by the information contained in this book or the use of any products mentioned. Readers should not use any of the products discussed in this book without the advice of a medical professional.

Library of Congress Cataloging-in-Publication Data

Rinzler, Carol Ann.
    The healing power of soy: the enlightened person's guide to nature's
wonder food / Carol Ann Rinzler.
        p.   cm.
    Includes index.
    ISBN 0-7615-1471-6
    1. Soybean—Therapeutic use.   2. Soyfoods—Therapeutic use.   3. Cookery
(Soybeans).   4. Menopause—Diet therapy.   5. Women—Health and hygiene.
    I. Title.
RM666.S59R56   1998
615'.32374—dc21   98-33576
                                                                              CIP

98 99 00 01 02 DD 10 9 8 7 6 5 4 3 2 1

Printed in the United States of America

How to Order

Single copies may be ordered from Prima Publishing, P.O. Box 1260BK, Rocklin, CA 95677; telephone (916) 632-4400. Quantity discounts are also available. On your letterhead, include information concerning the intended use of the books and the number of books you wish to purchase.

Visit us online at www.primahealth.com

Contents

7   Cooking with Soy   **121**

Preface

Five years ago, when I wrote *Estrogen and Breast Cancer: A Warning to Women,* there was already a growing list of well-designed scientific studies showing that excessive exposure to estrogen—whether it is the estrogen produced naturally in your body or the estrogen you take as birth control pills or hormone-replacement therapy—can increase the risk of breast cancer.

Today there are even more convincing studies, and many of the scientists and journalists who downplayed the risks of estrogen back in the early 1990s have lately been writing books and articles of their own, warning against the unwarranted use of hormones.

Nevertheless, as millions of baby boomers head for menopause and the potentially unpleasant effects of a natural decline in estrogen secretion, they are likely to worry more about estrogen deprivation than about estrogen excess. Absent a safe substitute, these women, like their mothers before them, may start hormone-replacement therapy, with its promise of eternal youth—not to mention relief from such mundane problems as dry skin and thinning hair.

That's why I am writing this book.

In September 1996, a major event occurred in the world of nutritional medicine: The Second International Symposium on the Role of Soy in Preventing and Treating Chronic Disease was convened in Brussels. Under the direction of Mark Messina, a pioneer in the field of soy research (formerly at the National Institutes of Health), dozens of nutrition scientists delivered groundbreaking reports on the healing powers of the simple soybean.

I first read about the conference while tooling around the Internet. Those of you who surf the Net know that wandering through cyberspace can be a mesmerizing experience. You start out looking for information on, say, cookbooks, and you wind up reading about yaks in the Himalayas without knowing quite how you got there.

In any event, what I read on-screen about the agenda at the conference in Brussels was so exciting that I immediately called Dr. Messina. He was kind enough to send to me a copy of the proceedings, a collection of papers about a food that, until I read through the Brussels reports, I had regarded as, well, boring.

No more. What the epidemiologists and researchers had gathered to say about the soybean and its ability to influence human health was a revelation. Not only do soyfoods apparently protect your heart and reduce your risk of some kinds of cancer, they may also strengthen your bones and, wonder of wonders, actually reduce the severity of hot flashes. In other words, it's possible that soybeans may offer a safe and effective alternative to menopausal hormone-replacement therapy.

Using the Brussels research and a plethora of additional studies and statistics, I hope to provide the information you need to decide whether soy foods will work for you. I'll begin with a brief biography of the definitely not-so-common soybean. Chapter One describes the basic nutrients in the bean—vitamins, minerals, proteins, fats, carbohydrates, and fiber—and explains how to integrate soybeans into your daily diet. Chapter Two details the nature of phytoestrogens, the fascinating family of natural chemicals that may deliver the benefits of estrogen with fewer risks.

This nutritional primer is followed by four chapters about the health benefits of soybeans. Many of these benefits specifically pertain to women undergoing menopause. At first, I couldn't decide whether to begin with the most common menopausal annoyance, the hot flash, or to go straight for heart disease, the leading killer of older women. In the end, the choice was clear: heart disease. Next comes a chapter on soy as a natural cancer-fighter, then a chapter about how soy builds better bones, and, finally, everything you ever wanted to know about how to cool a hot flash with—what else?—soy.

The last chapter is a brief but tasty collection of cooking tips and recipes for individual soy products: soybeans, tofu, tempeh, texturized soy protein, soy flours, soy milk, soy sauces, soybean oil, and miso. For the health-conscious couch potato, Appendix A offers a list of mail-order companies that will send soy products right to your door when you dial up their 800-numbers. Appendix B is a list of companies that manufacture and distribute soy products nationwide. Appendix C is a list of addresses for most of the researchers whose work is cited in this book.

I would also like to add a personal note of appreciation to Jamie Miller, my editor at Prima; Debra Venzke, my patient, painstaking project editor; my agent, Phyllis Westberg; and my husband, Perry Luntz, each of whom helped make this book a reality.

As you read through it, remember that the scientific version of the adage "there's no such thing as a free lunch" is "there's no remedy without risk." Right now, we know that the estrogenic compounds in soy are weaker and theoretically less problematic than the natural estrogens our bodies manufacture or than the synthetic estrogens we get from hormone drugs. For most people, there is very little doubt that the amount of phytoestrogens in soybeans are safe and that the soybean is a healthful food. The sole concern is whether high concentrations of phytoestrogens are safe for women who have already had breast cancer, are at risk for breast cancer, or have gone through menopause and have very low levels of natural estrogens. If you fall into one of these categories, you'll want to talk with your own doctor to see if she has any new information to add to the debate.

One thing more. While the science of soybeans is impressive, the beans are also good food. As epidemiologists continue to document the medical benefit of soybeans, I hope you will discover on your own what I found out while writing this book. Soybeans aren't only good for you—they taste good, too. Enjoy!

Introduction

Not Your Ordinary Bean

In the world of legumes, the soybean is an unlikely star. It isn't sleek and glossy like the black bean. It lacks the broad-shouldered muscle of the lima. There's none of the down-home warmth of the split pea, or the snap of a kidney bean in chili, or even the slightly musty flavor of chickpeas mashed in olive oil.

No, the soybean is just a bean, small, oval, beige, with no flavor to speak of, a culinary chameleon that takes on the characteristics of any food it's near. Mix it with eggs, and it tastes like eggs. Stir it into tomatoes, and that's what you'll taste. Combine it with ground chuck, and, presto! it's a beef-burger.

But Mother Nature loves surprises, and in creating the soybean, she has handed us a doozy. Right now, the unassuming legume is front and center on the medical stage, drawing rave reviews as study after study attests to its healthful brilliance.

Like other beans, the soybean is rich in fiber, low in sodium, and a powerhouse of B vitamins and iron. But that's just the beginning of its virtues. Unlike the protein in other veggies, including other beans, the soybean's proteins are complete, containing sufficient amounts of all the amino acids that are essential to human health. In other words, soy protein is the equivalent of protein from animal foods such as meat, poultry, fish, and dairy products.

Other beans do little nutritionally for your bones, but eating soybeans can actually make your bones stronger by enhancing your absorption of calcium. What's more, certain soy foods, such as enriched soy milk, are themselves calcium-rich. Other beans are practically fat-free. That's good. But the high-fat soybean yields an oil that is packed with heart-healthy monounsaturated and polyunsaturated fatty acids. That's different—and it's also good.

Best of all, the soybean is brimming with phytoestrogens, natural plant chemicals that seem to fight cancer, protect your heart, build bone density, and alleviate the signs of menopause.

In short, the humble soybean is Nature's Wonder Bean.

THE FIRST SOYBEANS

The earliest written record mentioning the soybean dates back to 2838 B.C. in China. After that, there's a l-o-o-o-n-g gap in the story, about a millennium and a half, until sometime around 1500 B.C., when a pair of rogues named Yu Xi-ong and Gong Gangshi turned up lost in a northern China desert with nothing to eat except the pea-like fruit of a previously unknown plant: the soybean.

These men, who were either bandits or warlords, depending on who's telling the story, must have been two tough hombres to survive on naked soybeans. While the bean is a veritable package of goodies—proteins, carbohydrates, fat, fiber, B vitamins, iron, and calcium—it is totally indigestible when eaten raw. Worse yet, the uncooked soybean contains chemicals that inactivate vital enzymes in your body (the chemicals are themselves inactivated when the beans are cooked). So you can assume that if Yu Xi-ong and Gong Gangshi survived on soybeans, they not only discovered the bean but were also the world's first soy chefs.

Fast forward a few hundred years, and you find the Chinese setting another milestone as they become the first people to cultivate the bean from the northern desert. They used the bean as animal fodder, as well as food for human beings. And here's a bonus: Growing soybeans improved the health and viability of the farm soil in China.

The Chinese were almost certainly the first people to create the most famous soybean product, the bean curd known as "tofu." You can bet that they invented tofu, around 200 B.C., by accident, which is not an unusual occurrence in the history of food. For example, the first yogurt probably materialized somewhere in north Africa when a householder left a pot of milk untended in the warm air, allowing bacteria that was floating by to land on the milk, digest its sugars into lactic acid, sour the milk, and produce a tangy, acidic, soured-milk product.

As for tofu, we can imagine that it was created something like this: Soybeans were often stored in seawater, to soften and preserve them. Saltwater is more dense than the liquid inside the beans, so a natural osmotic process took place, with milky liquid from the beans flowing out through the beans' "skin" into the water where it curdled (solidified) into the white food we call tofu.

By the 1600s, the Europeans, who had already appropriated spices from the East, as well as chocolate, yams, potatoes, and tomatoes from the vast new grocery store known as the New World, were beginning to cultivate soybean plants imported from China. Soybeans made their way to the United States in the early 1800s, but not as food: Sailors used them as ballast to balance the ships returning empty from trading in Asian ports.

Soon enough, the Brits and their American cousins began to enshrine the soybean and its bounty in verse. For example, here's a nifty little limerick from Edward Lear's *Book of Nonsense* (1862):

There was an old person of Troy,
Whose drink was warm brandy and soy,
Which he took from a spoon,
By the light of the moon,
In sight of the City of Troy.

Unlike tofu, soy sauce—the soy in the Lear jingle—was not an accidental discovery. According to the author of *Meals Medicinal*, an early (1896) collection of odd facts about the health power of food,

The beans are boiled, then mixed with barley, or wheat, until, through fermentation, they become covered with mold. Then brine is added, and further fermentation goes on for a couple of years. The sauce then concocted is afterward boiled afresh, and put, when cool, into bottles, or casks.

Or was there another way to make this exotic, intensely salty sauce that was so shocking to the Victorian palate, nourished on bland porridge and vegetables that were matter-of-factly boiled into mush? Rumor said yes, alluding to the dark possibility that soy sauce was made of (yuck!) black beetles. In this case, folklore and rumor were at least slightly connected to fact. According to J. Timbs, a contributor to *Popular Fallacies Explained and Corrected*, a 1924 collection of myths and rumors, this one's no exception. "The Chinese at Canton have a large soy manufactory," he writes, "and they are particularly solicitous to obtain cockroaches from ships." British sailors who were watching the Chinese concluded that the black cockroaches were used to make the black sauce, but, in fact, said Timbs, the Chinese used the bugs as fish bait. One British sea captain begged to disagree, noting that an "infusion" of cockroaches mixed with sea water did taste suspiciously like soy sauce. This led Timbs to wonder: How did the captain know?

Today, the soybean is the world's most commonly eaten plant, a dietary staple whose derivatives—proteins, fiber, flours, and oils—are used in manufactured foods in virtually every country on Earth. The United States, whose first beans came in as ballast, grows more than half (51%) of the world's soybeans, followed by Brazil (19%), Argentina (10%), China (8%), Paraguay (2%), and the European countries (1%).

Are you a numbers freak? Then here's a whopper for you: According to the United Soybean Board, a trade group representing soybean growers in the United States, the 2.5 billion bushels of soybeans grown each year in this country are enough to cover every inch of ground in every single one of the 50 states 255 times.

Soybean oils—used in our mayonnaise, margarines, salad dressings, and vegetable shortenings—account for 79% of all the edible fats and oils consumed each year in the United States. Soy flours, the simplest form of soy protein additives, are found in a wide variety of delicious commercial baked goods, noodles, mixes, frozen desserts, and instant milk drinks. Soy isolates, another form of protein additive, are found in imitation dairy products such as processed cheeses and coffee whiteners. Soy concentrates add texture and protein to soup bases, gravies, and protein "power drinks." Texturized soy protein, made from soy flour, is a no-cholesterol meat extender and a vegetarian meat substitute.

And if that isn't enough to convince you of the soybean's versatility, consider this. Soybeans may eventually power the bus that drives your kids to school. In December 1997, students at the Haines School in Medford, New Jersey (right smack in the middle of several hundred acres of soybeans, the leading field crop in the state—ahead of corn, wheat, hay, and potatoes), were the first to ride off in buses fueled with a mixture of soybean oil and diesel fuel. Over the next few years, under a $110,000 grant from the Federal Department of Energy, engineers will compare how these buses perform and whether they emit fewer noxious fumes than buses using regular fuel. The soy fuel, which burns cleaner than regular gas but costs about 60 cents more per gallon, has nonetheless already pulled in favorable reviews. "It smells like french fries or popcorn," said one fifth-grade participant in the test project.

HOW TO TALK SOY

The modern soybean is virtually a mother-of-invention, a parent to an entire family of what might fairly be called "classic designer foods." Throughout this book, you'll find references to many of these products, so before we jump into the pool of nutrition information, let's take a minute to define the various soyfoods. In alphabetical order they are

Miso: a thick salty paste made from soybeans, salt, and a mold culture that ferments the beans.

Soybean oil: the liquid fat that is extracted from soybeans; it is low in saturated fatty acids and high in polyunsaturates and monounsaturates.

Soy concentrates: a moderately high-protein (65%), high-fiber, moisturizing product that is used to add texture and protein to soy beverages, soup bases, and gravies.

Soy flour: a fine powder made by grinding roasted soybeans.

Soy isolates: a high-protein (90%), dry, fiber-free, carbohydrate-free product that is used to add texture to meat products or smoothness to processed cheeses and dairy substitutes such as coffee whiteners.

Soy milk: a thick white liquid made from ground soybeans or soy flour mixed with water.

Soy "nuts": roasted, whole, cooked beans.

Soy sauce (shoyu, tamari, teriyaki): salty liquids extracted from aged soybeans, or aged soybeans and wheat, mixed with a fermenting agent such as yeast plus (optional) seasonings.

Tempeh: a dense, chewy, fermented product made of whole, cooked soybeans combined with a thickening culture.

Texturized soy protein (TSP): granules or strips formed from soy flour. TSP is used as a chewy meat extender or meat substitute.

Tofu: a bland, cheese-like food made from the liquid squeezed out of soybeans. The liquid is stiffened with a coagulant, or "firming agent," such as gluconolactone or calcium chloride. Tofu made with a calcium coagulant is a good source of calcium.

There's one more word that crops up in almost every book about beans: *legume.* In fact, it's right there in the first sentence of this chapter. According to my Webster's *New Collegiate Dictionary*, a legume is "the fruit or seed of a pod-bearing plant (as peas or beans), [and so forth]." In other words, it's a family name for beans and peas, including the ubiquitous peanut. Frankly, I think it's much less pretentious just to write "beans" or "beans and peas." But who am I to argue with generations of cooks and cookbook writers?

1

The Nutritional Wonder Bean

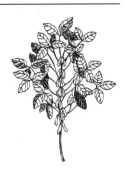

VITAMINS

When it comes to vitamins, you can spell soybeans' benefits with a capital "B" for the entire B family: riboflavin (vitamin B_1), thiamine (vitamin B_2), niacin, vitamin B_6 (sometimes listed as "pyridoxine" on supplement labels), folate (folic acid), and lecithin. (Soybeans are among the best food sources of lecithin. Other good sources are eggs, liver, wheat germ, and peanuts.)

The B vitamins are vital for human health and growth. They protect your appetite and make it possible for you to extract energy from food. They keep your skin and mucous membranes (the pink tissue lining your nose, throat, and other body cavities) in tip-top shape.

Soy foods can also be an unexpected source of vitamin B_{12}, a nutrient that we ordinarily get only from meat, fish, or poultry, or as a waste product created by bacteria that naturally live in our digestive tracts. Some soy milks are fortified with vitamin B_{12}, and the organisms that ferment soy sauces and tempeh produce vitamin B_{12}, which means that these foods are a good vegetarian source of the nutrient.

The current star of the B family is folate (sometimes identified as folic acid). When taken by a woman who is pregnant or trying to become pregnant, folate is so effective at reducing the risk of neural tube (spinal cord) birth defects that the U.S. government now requires supplement manufacturers to include 400 mcg of folate, more than twice the current RDA, in all multivitamin products.

1

In the spring of 1998, yet another health benefit for folate was revealed. Eric B. Rimm, M.D., of the Harvard School of Public Health, analyzed data from a survey of the records for more than 80,000 women enrolled in the long-running Nurses Health Study at Harvard School of Public Health/Brigham and Woman's Hospital in Boston and identified the first direct link between two B vitamins and the health of the heart. According to Dr. Rimm, consuming a diet that provides more than 400 mcg of folate and 3 mg of vitamin B_6 a day from either food or supplements, which is more than twice the current RDA for each, may reduce a woman's risk of heart attack by almost 50%. (For more about folate's ability to protect your heart, see Chapter Three, "Soy and Your Heart.")

Right now, no similar evidence exists to prove the benefits of B vitamins for men. But here's another bit of news to chew on. In his analysis, Dr. Rimm also identified something else that contributes to heart health: moderate amounts of alcohol. Adding one drink a day to the folate-and-B_6 banquet appears to increase a woman's protection, lowering her risk of heart attack by nearly 80%. For the record, one drink equals 1 ounce of spirits, 5 ounces of wine, or 12 ounces of beer.

Recommendations for B Vitamins

The simplest guide to safe and effective doses for all nutrients is the list of Recommended Dietary Allowances (RDA) created by the Food and Nutrition Board of the National Research Council. As you probably know, the RDAs are simply protective recommendations designed to prevent your developing a nutritional deficiency; they are not recommendations for optimum health.

Today, many nutrition scientists are taking a new look at the RDAs. Many recent well-designed studies and re-analyses of existing data (such as the information from the Nurses Health Study regarding folate and vitamin B_6) make it clear that doses larger than the RDAs may be beneficial, either as a lifetime requirement or at times when people are experiencing situations that subject them to additional stress.

The trick is to obtain the nutrients you need without straying into potentially hazardous mega-dose territory. For example, while

Table 1-1 Recommended Dietary Allowances (RDA) for B Vitamins
for Healthy Adults

	Thiamine mg	Riboflavin mg	Niacin mg	Vitamin B_6 mg	Folate mcg	Vitamin B_{12} mcg
Women (age)						
19–24	1.1	1.3	15	1.6	180	2.0
25–50	1.1	1.3	15	1.6	180	2.0
51+	1.0	1.2	13	1.6	180	2.0
Men (age)						
19–24	1.5	1.7	19	2.0	200	2.0
25–50	1.5	1.7	19	2.0	200	2.0
51+	1.2	1.4	15	2.0	200	2.0

Source: National Research Council, *Recommended Dietary Allowances* (Washington,
D.C.: National Academy Press, 1989).

Dr. Rimm's examination of the Nurses Health Study implies that a
daily intake of folate and vitamin B_6 that is twice the current RDA
may help prevent birth defects and reduce the risk of heart attack,
very high daily doses of vitamin B_6, in the gram range (more than
1,000 to 2,000 mg), have been linked to temporary nerve damage.

As a nutrition-savvy consumer, you will want to stay tuned for
more on the soy-and-vitamin-B story. Meanwhile, Table 1-1 lists the
current RDAs for B vitamins for healthy adults (men and women
ages 19 and older).

Getting B Vitamins from Soy Foods

Okay, so now you know that B vitamins are especially valuable in
protecting your heart and your reproductive health and that soy
foods are a good source of B vitamins. Next question: Exactly how
many soybeans do you have to eat to get the Bs you need? Answer:
Table 1-2 lists the amounts of five different B vitamins in a standard

Table 1-2 The B Vitamins in Soy Foods

Food 3.5 oz/100 grams*	Thiamine mg	Riboflavin mg	Niacin mg	Vitamin B_6 mg	Folate mcg
Miso	0.10	0.25	0.86	0.22	33.0
Natto	0.16	0.19	0	n/a	n/a
Soy flour					
defatted	0.70	0.25	2.61	0.57	305.4
full fat	0.58	1.16	4.52	0.46	345.0
Soy sauce	0.06	0.15	3.95	0.20	18.2
Soybeans					
boiled	0.16	0.29	0.40	0.23	55.8
roasted	0.10	0.15	1.41	0.21	211.0
Soy milk	0.16	0.07	0.15	0.04	1.5
Tempeh	0.13	0.11	4.63	0.30	52.0
Tofu (firm)	0.16	0.10	0.38	0.09	29.3

*about ½ cup

Source: USDA, *Composition of Foods,* USDA Handbook #8-16 (Washington, D.C.).

serving (3.5 ounces/100 grams/about ½ cup) of several different soy foods.

MINERALS

All beans are low in sodium and rich in heart-healthy potassium, bone-building calcium and phosphorus, plus iron and magnesium. Yet here, as in so many other areas of nutrition, the soybean is definitely a cut above the rest.

Ounce for ounce, soybeans give you up to two or three times the calcium, phosphorus, iron, and magnesium you get from other popular beans. Better yet, while the calcium and iron in other plant foods are often bound into compounds that your body has difficulty digesting and absorbing, the calcium and iron in tofu made with a calcium stiffener are readily available. Calcium-fortified soy milks are available but have not been evaluated with respect to their calcium absorption. For example, your body finds it three times easier to extract and use the iron from tofu than it does the iron from any other bean or bean food, including tofu's parent, the soybean itself. As Dr. Mark Andon has written in *Super Calcium Miracle: The Calcium Citrate Malate Breakthrough* (also from Prima Publishing), "One to 1.5 servings of calcium-set tofu will yield the absorbable calcium in a glass of milk."

To put that into practical terms, if you are a healthy adult, ages 25 to 51, you can obtain nearly 25% of your RDA for calcium, 59% to 88% of your RDA for iron, 42% to 56% of your RDA for magnesium, and 13% to 17% of your RDA for zinc from a single 3.5-ounce serving, about ½ cup, of cooked soybeans. Note: The RDAs for iron, magnesium, and zinc are higher for men than for women, so when you see a range, such as 58% to 88% of the RDA for iron, the lower number represents the percentage of the RDA for men, the higher number, the percentage of the RDA for women.

How many beans do you need to get the minerals you require? Table 1-3 compares the mineral content of a standard 3.5-ounce/100-gram serving of several different kinds of plain cooked beans.

Table 1-3 The Mineral Content of a Standard Serving of Several Different Kinds of Beans

Bean 3.5 oz/100 g	Calcium mg	Phosphorus mg	Iron mg	Sodium mg	Potassium mg	Magnesium mg	Zinc mg
Soybeans	175.44	421.4	8.84	1.72	885.8	147.92	1.98
Black beans	46.44	240.8	3.61	1.71	810.6	120.4	1.93
Chick-peas	61.2	212.5	2.55	8.5	455.6	73.1	1.72
Kidney beans	49.56	251.34	5.2	3.54	713.31	79.65	1.89
Lentils	37.62	356.4	6.59	3.96	730.62	71.28	2.51
Split peas	27.44	194.04	2.53	3.92	709.52	70.56	1.96

Source: USDA, *Composition of Foods*, USDA Handbook #8-16 (Washington, D.C.).

PROTEINS

Proteins are an essential nutrient composed of small units called amino acids ("the building blocks of proteins") linked together in "chains" to form very long molecules. They are found in every cell of your body and in the deoxyribonucleic acid (DNA) in the cell nucleus that carries your genetic inheritance.

Your body uses proteins to build cells, maintain healthy tissues, and create other specialized proteins called enzymes that enable your body to perform the hundreds of individual functions you simply take for granted in a normal life: moving, breathing, thinking, seeing, hearing, digesting food, and so on.

The Different Kinds of Proteins in Food

To make the proteins that our bodies require, we human beings need 22 different amino acids. Nine of them are called "essential" because we cannot manufacture them in our bodies; we have to get them directly from food. The other 13 are called "nonessential," not because we don't need them, but because we can build them ourselves from the 9 essential amino acids. Table 1-4 lists the essential and nonessential amino acids for human beings.

All protein foods contain every amino acid listed in Table 1-4. The important question is, how much of each essential amino acid does the food contain? Foods with sufficient amounts of the essential amino acids are called foods with complete proteins. Foods lacking sufficient amounts of the essential amino acids are said to have incomplete or limited proteins.

An animal's body is very like ours, so foods from animals—meat, fish, poultry, milk, and eggs—are good sources of complete proteins. Plants, on the other hand, often have limited amounts of one or more of the essential amino acids. That's why grains, fruit, vegetable, nuts, and seeds are said to deliver limited or incomplete proteins.

Nutritionists know that you can improve the quality of the proteins you ingest from plants, either by eating plant foods with animal foods or by eating two or more different plant foods, with differing amounts of various amino acids, at the same time or in the same dish. For example, grains (pasta) are low in the essential amino acids lysine and isoleucine, which are abundant in dairy foods (cheese). So

Table 1-4 Amino Acids for Human Beings

Essential Amino Acids

Phenylalanine	Lysine
Isoleucine	Methionine
Threonine	Leucine
Tryptophane	Valine
Histadine	

Nonessential Amino Acids

Alanine	Arginine
Asparagine	Aspartic acid
Cysteine	Cystine
Glutamic acid	Glutamine
Glycine	Hydroxyproline
Proline	Serine
Tyrosine	

---

macaroni and cheese is not simply a tasty treat; it's a nutritionally valid way to make sure you get the amino acids you need. The same thing applies to the classic peanut butter and jelly sandwich. The bread (grain) supplies the amino acids missing from the nuts (peanut butter), and vice versa. The jelly, which plays no part in this nutritional partnership, is an optional pleasure. Putting foods together to make a combination with the right amount of amino acids is called "completing." The amino acids in the cheese and those in the pasta complete the proteins in the dish. Ditto for bread and peanut butter.

Table 1-5 shows several ways to combine different kinds of food so as to complete their proteins.

The Special Protein Power of Soy

When it comes to protein, soy is unique among the plant foods. While other vegetables (including other beans), grains, and fruits have incomplete, or limited, proteins, the proteins in soybeans are complete. They have sufficient amounts of all the essential amino

Table 1-5 Combining Foods to Make Complete Protein Dishes

Whole grains	+	beans and peas
Whole grains	+	meat, fish, poultry, or dairy products
Beans and peas	+	dairy products
Nuts and seeds	+	dairy products
Vegetables	+	meat, fish, poultry, or dairy foods

acids, a surprising attribute that more than justifies the Chinese description of tofu as "meat without bones."

Because of their unique composition, soy foods provide protein that is the equal of protein from animal foods. No, come to think of it, the soybean is actually a better protein food than meat, chicken, poultry, eggs, or milk. Those animal foods serve up their protein with cholesterol and lots of saturated fat. Soy foods deliver their protein cholesterol-free and low in saturated fats. As a result, getting your protein from animal foods can raise your cholesterol levels and may increase your risk of heart disease, while getting your protein from soy foods reduces your cholesterol levels and increases the health of your heart. (See Chapter Three, "Soy and Your Heart.")

How potent is the protein in soy? One easy way to find out is to rate it on the scale used by nutrition scientists to measure a food's protein quality as compared to the protein in egg whites, the food that is arbitrarily ranked 100 (sometimes written 1.0), meaning it is the easiest form of protein for your body to absorb and use. Table 1-6 ranks the protein availability of egg whites against the protein availability of seven other foods, including the protein in soybeans and two other kinds of beans. As you can see, the protein from the powerful soybean is right up there, on a par with egg white and casein, the protein in milk.

How Much Protein Do You Need?

Your age and whether you are a man or a woman play a large role in determining your daily protein requirements. As a general rule, young people need lots of protein to enable them to sustain their continuing rapid body growth. On average, men need more protein than women because the male body is larger and the male metabolism

Table 1-6 Comparing Proteins

Food	Protein Quality
Egg white	1.0
Isolated soy protein	1.0
Casein (milk protein)	1.0
Beef	.95*
Kidney beans (canned)	.70*
Lentils (canned)	.60*
Whole wheat flour	.40*
White flour	.36*

*Approximate

Source: United Soybean Board, Soy Facts #10, Soyfoods and Protein, (n.d.).

(the rate at which the body burns energy for basic tasks such as heart-beat and breathing) burns fuel faster, meaning that men need to take in more just to stay even.

As with vitamins and minerals, the simplest guide to your daily protein requirements are the National Research Council's Recommended Dietary Allowances. Table 1-7 shows the protein RDAs for healthy adults, ages 19 and older.

Table 1-7 Recommended Dietary Allowances (RDA) of Protein for Healthy Adults

Gender	Age	RDA (grams)
Women	19–24	58
	25–50	63
	51+	63
Men	19–24	72
	25–50	79
	51+	77

Source: National Research Council, *Recommended Dietary Allowances* (Washington, D.C.: National Academy Press, 1989).

Using Soy to Fill Your Protein Requirements

Substituting soy foods for other high-protein foods is easy once you know how much protein you get from a representative serving of a particular soy food. For example, you don't have to be a rocket scientist to know that you can substitute soy milk for cow's milk to get the cholesterol-free protein you need. Eight ounces of full-fat, but cholesterol-free, soy milk gives you 10 grams of protein; 8 ounces of fat-free, no-cholesterol soy milk has 7 grams of protein. Eight ounces of skim milk has more protein (8.35 grams) than fat-free soy milk, but it also has cholesterol.

Table 1-8 shows the protein content of common servings of lean ground beef, skim milk, and one whole egg versus the protein content of common servings of several soy products.

Stop! Read This Soy Protein Alert

Food allergy is an uncommon but potentially serious reaction to proteins in specific foods, including soybeans. Many people are sensitive

Table 1-8 Protein Content of Common Foods

Food	Serving	Protein (grams)
Lean ground beef	3 oz	21
Skim milk	8 oz	8.35
Whole egg (extra large)	1	7.2
Miso	2 tbsp	4
Soybeans (boiled)	½ cup	14
Soy flour		
full-fat	½ cup	15
low-fat	½ cup	21
Soy milk	½ cup	4
Soy protein isolate	½ cup	46
Tofu		
raw, firm	½ cup	20
raw, regular	½ cup	10
Tempeh	½ cup	16

Source: United Soybean Board, *The 5000-Year-Old Secret* (n.d.); USDA Handbook No. 8-16 (Washington, D.C.: USDA, 1986).

to the peanut, a plant that is related to beans. Others may react to soybeans or soy foods such as soy milk, soy sauce, tofu, and tempeh. If you are sensitive to soy, after eating a soy food you may experience irritated, swollen lips; stomach cramps; chills; or vomiting.

But here's an interesting medical fact. Sometimes people who react to a soy product are actually reacting to corn. They experience allergic problems after eating soy because the soy food may have been stored, or handled, or carried in a container previously used for corn. The minute amount of corn residue in the container is enough to trigger an allergic reaction. A similar situation may occur when people who are sensitive to peanuts consume chocolates prepared in the same factory as peanuts.

If you think you may be sensitive to soy products, don't guess. Check with your doctor who can administer tests that will identify the allergy or rule it out.

FATS

Despite continuing bad publicity, dietary fats and oils are important to our health. We need the fats that we get from food for energy, to build cells and tissues, as insulation for our nerves, to synthesize hormones and other biochemicals, and to make the layers and pads of fat that cushion our organs, protect us against the cold, and, of course, round out our shape.

The Different Kinds of Dietary Fats

Nutritionists describe dietary fats and oils in terms of their basic components, molecules of fatty acids. There are three kinds of fatty acids: saturated fatty acids, polyunsaturated fatty acids, and monounsaturated fatty acids. Butter, which contains more saturated than unsaturated fatty acids, is called a saturated fat. Safflower oil, which contains more polyunsaturated fatty acids than saturated or monounsaturated ones, is called a polyunsaturated oil. Canola oil, which contains more monounsaturated than saturated or polyunsaturated fatty acids, is called a monounsaturated oil.*

---

*A dietary fat is called a fat when it is hard, like butter, and an oil when it's liquid, like safflower oil.

Table 1-9 Comparing the Fatty Acid Content of Dietary Oils

	Fatty Acids		
Fat/Oil	Saturated	Polyunsaturated	Monounsaturated
Canola oil	6%	36%	58%
Safflower oil	9%	78%	13%
Corn oil	13%	62%	25%
Olive oil	14%	9%	77%
Soybean oil	15%	67%	24%
Peanut oil	18%	34%	48%
Cottonseed oil	27%	54%	19%
Palm oil	51%	10%	39%
Palm kernel oil	86%	2%	12%
Coconut oil	92%	2%	6%

Source: United Soybean Board, *Soybeans: Unlocking the Secret to Good Nutrition* (St. Louis, Mo., n.d.).

Some dietary fats and oils are clearly less beneficial than others. Saturated fats, found most abundantly in foods of animal origin, are hazardous to your heart. They raise your cholesterol level and increase your risk of heart attack. Polyunsaturated fatty acids and monounsaturated fatty acids, which are abundant in plant foods, are protective. They reduce cholesterol levels and lower the risk of heart disease. Table 1-9 compares the fatty acid content of several dietary oils.

The Fats in Soybeans

The soybean's fats are as unusual as its protein. Unlike other beans, which derive less than 14% of their calories from fat, the soybean may get more than 40% of its calories from fats. For example, a 3.5-ounce/100-gram serving of kidney beans has 127 calories, 92 calories from carbohydrates, 36 from protein, and less than 9 from fat. The same size serving of soybeans has 189 calories, including 40 from carbohydrates, 68 from protein, and a whopping 81 from fats. If fats are bad, how can that be good? Because it's the whole package that counts, and when everything is added up, the soybean is still a nutritional bargain.

Soybean oil has no cholesterol. It is low in saturated fatty acids and high in unsaturated ones. It is a good source of two essential fatty acids, linoleic acid and linolenic acid, which, like the essential amino acids (see the earlier section, "Proteins"), must be obtained from food because we cannot synthesize them from other fatty acids. And soybean oil is rich in omega-3 fatty acids. Omega-3s, also found in fish such as salmon, are believed to reduce the risk of heart disease and may help keep our bones strong (see Chapter Five, "Building Better Bones with Soy"). Finally, soybean oil is well stocked with monounsaturated fatty acids, including oleic acid, which may actually *lower* cholesterol levels.

How Soybeans Balance a Healthful Diet

When dealing with dietary fat, the trick is to get what you need and no more. According to the Dietary Guidelines for Americans created by the U.S. Department of Agriculture and the Department of Health and Human Services, an optimally healthful diet derives no more than 30% of its total calories from fat and no more than 10% of its total calories from saturated fats. (The calories from saturated fats are counted in the total calories from fat.)

Let's translate that into real-life terms. If you consume about 2,000 calories a day, a typical American diet, you should get no more than 600 of those calories from fat, and no more than 200 calories from saturated fats. Remember: Your total saturated fat allowance is part of your total fat intake, not added to it. If your 2,000 calorie diet allows 600 fat calories a day, 200 of those may be from saturated fats; 400 should come from unsaturated fats.

Table 1-10 calculates the amount of fat and saturated fat calories that constitute the recommended intake at several levels of the day's total calories.

Soybeans and soy products, which are low in saturated fats, can easily be used as substitutes for meats and other animal foods. For example, texturized soy protein (TSP) granules are available in many health food stores. As you can see from Table 1-11, using these granules to replace 30% of the ground meat in a typical lasagna recipe

Table 1-10 Examples of Recommended Consumption of Fats As a Percentage of Total Daily Calories

Total Daily Calories	Total Fat Calories (% of Total Daily Calories) 30%	Saturated Fat Calories (% of Total Daily Calories) 10%
1,500	450	150
2,000	600	200
2,500	750	250
3,000	900	300

serves up the same high-protein meal while reducing the total fat content per portion by 36%, the saturated fat content by 33%, and the cholesterol content by 31%. Not a bad bargain.

You can make similar substitutions with other soy foods using the information in Table 1-12, which compares the total fat and saturated fat content of common foods and their soy alternatives.

CARBOHYDRATES

There are two kinds of carbohydrates: simple ones and complex ones. Both are composed of one or more units of sugar. What distinguishes one type from the other is how many units of sugar they contain.

Table 1-11 Comparing Recipes: All-Meat Lasagna versus Lasagna with Soy

	All-Meat Lasagna	Soy Lasagna
Total fat	10.7 grams	6.9 grams
Saturated fat	4.5 grams	3.0 grams
Cholesterol	71.0 mg	49.0 mg
Protein	19.0 grams	19.0 grams

Source: United Soybean Board, *Talk Soy.*

Table 1-12 Fat Content of Soy Foods

Food (amount)	Total Fat (grams)	Saturated Fat (grams)
Lean ground beef, broiled (3 oz)	13.9	5.5
Soybeans, boiled (½ cup)	7.7	1.1
Tempeh (½ cup)	6.4	0.9
Tofu, raw, firm (½ cup)	11.0	1.5
Whole wheat flour (½ cup)	1.1	0.2
White flour (½ cup)	0.6	0.1
Soy flour, defatted (½ cup)	0.5	0.0
Soy flour, full-fat (½ cup)	8.6	1.2
Whole milk (1 cup)	8.2	5.1
Skim milk (1 cup)	0.4	0.3
Soy milk (1 cup)	2.3	0.2

Source: United Soybean Board, *The 5,000-Year-Old Secret* (n.d.). USDA Handbook No. 8-16 (Washington, D.C.: USDA, 1986).

A simple carbohydrate, such as fructose (the sugar in fruit), glucose (the form of sugar found in our blood), or galactose (milk sugar), has one unit of sugar. A complex carbohydrate, such as sucrose (table sugar) or raffinose (a carbohydrate in soybeans), has two or more units of sugar. Dietary fiber, such as the gums hemicellulose and cellulose in soybeans, is a complex carbohydrate composed of either many units of sugar or many units of sugar plus chemicals (called uronic acids) that are derived from other sugars.

The soybean's protein is unusual and so is its fat content, but its carbohydrates are strictly "by the book." In other words, like other beans, the soybean is packed to the brim with carbs.

The Complex Carbohydrates in Soybeans

The two most important sugars in soybeans are the complex carbohydrates raffinose and stachyose. Raffinose is a three-unit molecule with one unit each of galactose, glucose, and fructose. Stachyose is a four-unit molecule with one unit each of glucose and fructose, plus two units of galactose.

Human beings have a hard time digesting raffinose and stachyose. When these sugars reach our digestive tract, they tend to sit there, forming a banquet for the resident bacteria who chomp away on the sugars, releasing as waste the gas that makes us uncomfortable after eating beans. Soaking beans before you cook them pulls raffinose and stachyose out into the water. Discard the soaking water and you reduce the amount of indigestible sugar in the beans, which means they are now less likely to give you gas.

In addition to raffinose and stachyose, soybeans are a good source of the complex carbohydrates we call fiber. Like other beans, soy contains gums, the soluble fiber that dissolves in your stomach to produce a gel that is believed to carry cholesterol and fats out of your body. This is the basis for the theory that a diet rich in beans and peas, as well as in other gum-rich foods, lowers your risk of heart disease.

Soybeans also provide insoluble fibers, the indigestible lignin, cellulose, and hemicellulose in seed coverings that exert a laxative action, carrying food more quickly through your body. Insoluble fiber is believed to reduce the risk of colon cancer and help ward off or relieve such digestive disorders as constipation or diverticulosis, a condition characterized by pouches in the wall of the gut where trapped food may trigger an infection.

The currently recommended daily fiber intake is approximately 25 grams of total fiber (insoluble fiber and soluble fiber combined). Few Americans actually get this much fiber, but adding soybeans to your diet is a delicious way to increase your fiber consumption.

Table 1-13 lists the amount of total fiber in one 3.5-ounce/100-gram serving of several soy foods.

Soy's Complex Carbohydrates Help Control Diabetes

Foods high in complex carbohydrates are useful for people with diabetes because they are digested slowly, requiring less insulin (a hormone that aids digestion) than foods containing simple sugars. More than 90 years ago, British writer W. T. Fernie, M.D., author of such tomes as *Herbal Simples, Animal Simples,* and *Kitchen Physics,* wrote that beans were "an admirable substitute for bread in diabetes, a flour being prepared from them, and kneaded into loaves, or biscuits."

Table 1-13 The Fiber Content of Soy Foods

Food	Serving	Fiber (grams)*
Miso	2 tablespoons	1.9
Soy flour		
defatted	½ cup	7.7
full-fat	½ cup	4.1
Soybeans		
boiled	½ cup	5.4
roasted	½ cup	3.0
Soy milk	½ cup	1.6
Tofu		
firm	½ cup	0.2
regular	½ cup	1.5

*Soluble plus insoluble fiber
Source: United Soybean Board, *The 5000-Year-Old Secret* (n.d.).

Fernie thought that it was because beans were low in starch. Today we know it's because those complex carbohydrates, including starch, can be digested with relatively small amounts of insulin and thus produce only a gradual increase in blood sugar levels. In fact, a mid-1980s study at the University of Kentucky demonstrated that following a bean, whole grain, and vegetable diet that was developed at the University of Toronto may enable people with Type I diabetes (the form of the disease that results when the body produces virtually no insulin) to reduce their daily insulin injections by 38%. People with Type II diabetes, in which the body produces some insulin but not enough, are able to reduce their insulin injections by 98% on this diet.

FITTING SOY INTO YOUR DIET

As a food, soy's greatest virtue may be its versatility. No matter what your favorite foods are, there's likely to be a soy version you can slip into your daily diet. The easiest way to do this is to use the new food pyramids to plan your weekly menus.

The food pyramid is a relatively new device that was designed to simplify the task of putting together a balanced diet. At the pyramid's bottom is a broad base, representing foods you should eat every day. The middle shows foods you probably should include in your daily diet, but in smaller amounts than the foods at the bottom. The narrow, pointed top, represents food you should eat only once in a while or in very small amounts. The best lesson of the food pyramid is its visual depiction of the truism that good nutrition requires a variety of foods.

The U.S. Department of Agriculture created the first food pyramid in 1982 to replace an outdated guide, the Four Food Groups—vegetables and fruits, breads and cereals, milk and milk products, meat and meat alternatives such as beans. The foods in the four group plan are still valuable, of course, but the pyramid apportions them in a more modern manner that is designed to reduce the amount of high-fat, high-cholesterol foods obtained from animals. For example, the Four Food Group Plan listed fruits and vegetables together; the pyramid divides them into two separate groups. In addition, the pyramid calculates the number of servings you should get each day from each food category, that is, 6 to 11 servings of breads and other grain foods, with a lower number for people on a lower calorie (1,000) regimen and a higher number for people who consume as much as 3,000 calories a day.

Figure 1-1 shows the USDA food guide pyramid; Table 1-14 on page 20 explains what the USDA means when it says "one serving."

In 1993, a group of Boston-based nutritionists created a second food pyramid, the Mediterranean Diet Food Pyramid, to reflect the diet followed by people living in countries around the Mediterranean Sea. This diet is heavy on grains, fruits, and vegetables. Dairy products such as cheese and yogurt are used only as accents. There is practically no meat. The recommended fat is olive oil. And a glass of wine with meals is definitely on the menu. In other words, it's a low-cholesterol, low-fat, low-saturated fat, primarily vegetarian diet.

Like other high-plant, low-animal food regimens, the Mediterranean Food Pyramid is associated with a lower risk of heart disease and certain kinds of cancer. And like the USDA Food Guide Pyramid, it makes a clear statement about the value of variety at the

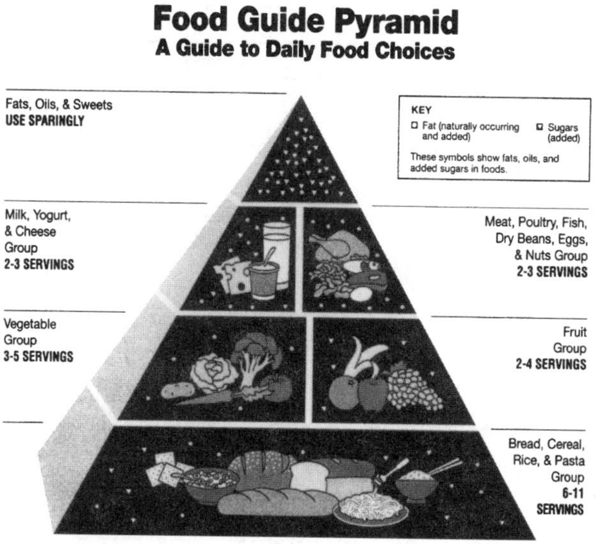

Food Guide Pyramid
A Guide to Daily Food Choices

Fats, Oils, & Sweets
USE SPARINGLY

KEY
□ Fat (naturally occurring   □ Sugars
and added)   (added)
These symbols show fats, oils, and
added sugars in foods.

Milk, Yogurt,
& Cheese
Group
2-3 SERVINGS

Meat, Poultry, Fish,
Dry Beans, Eggs,
& Nuts Group
2-3 SERVINGS

Vegetable
Group
3-5 SERVINGS

Fruit
Group
2-4 SERVINGS

Bread, Cereal,
Rice, & Pasta
Group
6-11
SERVINGS

Figure 1-1 The USDA Food Pyramid

table. But unlike the USDA version, the Mediterranean Diet Food Pyramid asks you to make your own decision about portions by looking at the guide and figuring out for yourself how to balance a plate (and a day).

Figure 1-2 on page 21 shows the Mediterranean Diet Food Pyramid.

Soy's Place on the Pyramids

What makes soybeans and soy products special is that, unlike most other foods, they fit easily into not one, not two, not three, not four, but five of the six basic food groups. First, soybeans are vegetables. They belong in the vegetable, or fruit and vegetable, group. Second, soybeans have complete proteins, so they fit into the "meat-fish-poultry" group. Third, some soy products, such as tofu made with a calcium thickener, are good sources of calcium and can be included in the milk and dairy foods group. Fourth, soy flours and soy grits work in the grains and cereal group. Fifth, soy oil is a natural for the fats, oils, and sweets group.

Table 1-14 One Serving on the USDA Food Pyramid

Food	One Serving
Bread, cereal, rice, pasta	1 slice bread 1 ounce of ready-to-eat cereal ½ cup of cooked cereal ½ cup of cooked rice or pasta
Vegetables	1 cup of raw leafy vegetables ½ cup of raw/cooked vegetables ¾ cup of vegetable juice
Fruits	1 medium piece of fresh fruit ½ cup of cooked fruit ¾ cup of fruit juice
Milk products	1 cup of milk or yogurt 1½ ounces of natural cheese 2 ounces of processed cheese
Meat, fish, poultry, dry beans, eggs, nuts, seeds	2 to 3 ounces of cooked lean meat or poultry or fish 1 egg or equivalent of egg substitute ½ cup of cooked dry beans ⅓ cup of nuts or seeds
Fats, oils, sweets	no set amount

Source: International Food Information Council Foundation, U.S. Department of Agriculture, Food Marketing Institute, The Food Guide Pyramid (Washington, D.C., 1995).

Table 1-15 lists servings of soy foods that are equivalent to other foods commonly used to satisfy the requirements of the food pyramids.

To show you how soybeans and soy foods fit in at every level of a healthful diet, the United Soybean Board has created its own food pyramid. Figure 1-3 on page 22 shows USB's Daily Soyfood Guide Pyramid.

SUMMING UP

The soybean is an unusual food, both highly nutritious and extraordinarily adaptable. Its prodigious supply of B vitamins puts it in the

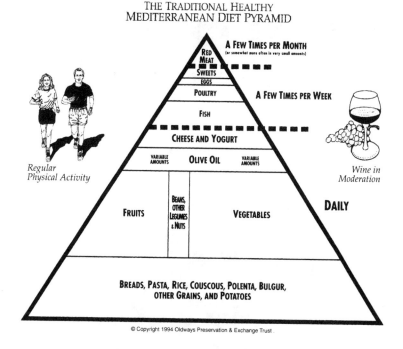

Figure 1-2 Mediterranean Diet Food Pyramid

Source: © 1994 Oldways Preservation and Exchange Trust. Reprinted by permission.

Table 1-15 Soy Food Servings Equal to One Serving of Common Foods

Soy Food	Common Food
1.5 cups of cooked soybeans	1 meat group serving
3-ounce soy burger	1 meat group serving
3 ounces of tofu	1 meat group serving
1 cup of soy milk or soy yogurt	1 milk group serving
½ cup of cooked soy grits	1 grain group serving
1 teaspoon of soy oil	1 teaspoon fat or oil

Source: United Soybean Board.

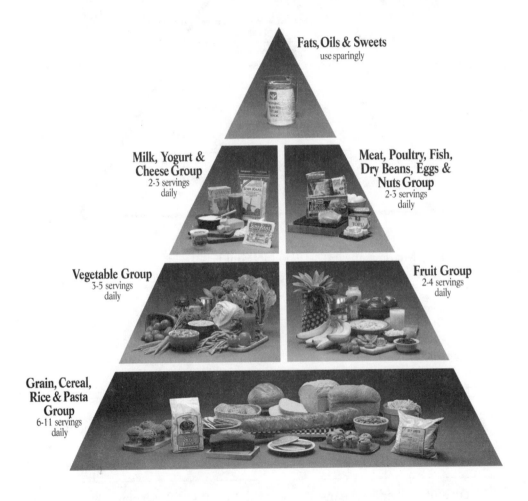

Figure 1-3 Daily Soyfood Guide Pyramid

Source: © United Soybean Board. Reprinted by permission.

front line of our nutritional defense against heart disease and birth defects. Its supply of minerals, specifically calcium, phosphorus, and magnesium, makes it a bone-builder. Soy's complete protein gives it a special place in the pantheon of vegetable meat-extenders and substitutes, and its carbohydrates ensure its value not only for people with diabetes but for those looking to reduce their risk of heart attack and certain kinds of cancer, such as cancer of the colon.

But soybeans have more to offer than their array of nutrients. They are also a treasure chest of phytoestrogens, chemical compounds in plants that behave like weaker versions of the estrogens we make in our own bodies or the synthetic estrogens we sometimes take as medicines. What makes phytoestrogens especially exciting is the possibility that they may deliver the benefits of estrogen without the risks.

And that is the story that begins in Chapter Two.

2

Something Special in the Bean

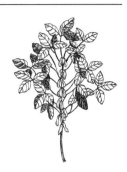

HORMONES AND PEOPLE AND PLANTS

All animals, including human beings, secrete natural chemicals called hormones, many of which belong to the chemical family known as steroids. The identifying feature of steroids is an arrangement of atoms in four circular patterns called "rings." (Other well-known chemicals that share the ring pattern are vitamin D and cholesterol.)

Our hormones regulate, influence, or change the behavior and sometimes even the structure of our body's organs and systems. Hormones make it possible for us to digest our food. They govern our growth. When we feel threatened, hormones quicken our heartbeat, tighten our muscles, and help us breathe faster so that we can think and move rapidly. When we are calm, hormones slow our heart rate and breathing, relax our muscles, and allow us to rest or sleep.

Table 2-1 lists some of the most important human hormones and shows their functions.

Every hormone we secrete has an important role to play in our bodies, but no role is more fascinating than that played by our sex hormones, estrogen and testosterone, which determine our gender, stimulate our sexual development, and maintain our reproductive organs and capabilities.

Estrogen and Testosterone

Both male bodies and female bodies secrete the two sex hormones, estrogen and testosterone. It is the ratio between the two, rather than

Table 2-1 Some Important Hormones in the Human Body

Hormone	Secreted By	Function
Adrenaline	adrenal glands	increases heart rate, constricts blood vessels, tightens muscles in the classic "fight or flight" reaction
Estrogen	ovaries	stimulates development of female sex characteristics, and maintains female reproductive health
Insulin	pancreas	assists in digestion
Secretin	gastric lining	triggers secretion of pancreatic juices for digestion
Somatotropin	pituitary gland	promotes and regulates growth
Testosterone	testes	stimulates development of male sex characteristics, maintains male reproductive health
Thyrotropin	hypophasis (hypothalamus gland)	stimulates growth and function of thyroid gland
Vasopressin	pituitary gland	controls contraction and relaxation of smooth muscle tissue, such as in the lining of the blood vessels and the uterus

Source: *Stedman's Medical Dictionary*, 26th Ed. (Baltimore, Md.: Williams & Wilkins, 1995).

the absence of one or the other, that makes us men or women. In other words, men have proportionately more testosterone; women, proportionately more estrogen.

The most important source of estrogen is the female ovary. Testosterone comes primarily from the testes. But thrifty Mother Nature, no fool she, has also arranged alternate sources of supply. If necessary, your body can synthesize sex hormones from chemicals that are secreted by glands other than the ovaries and testes or you can convert chemicals that are stored in other parts of your body to sex hormones.

Being able to make sex hormones from other naturally occurring biochemicals is a very useful skill. For example, after menopause, when a woman's ovaries secrete less estrogen, her body can still make estrogen from vitamin D, a steroid stored in fatty tissue under her skin, or from hormones secreted by the adrenal glands. The only difference is that while prior to menopause the most prevalent estrogen in a woman's body is estradiol, the form of estrogen secreted by the ovary, after menopause it is estrone, an estrogen produced by synthesis or conversion.

Unfortunately, for many women approaching menopause, this alternate supply of estrogen is not sufficient to prevent the discomforts associated with falling estrogen levels. To relieve hot flashes, mood swings, insomnia, vaginal irritation, or dry skin, these women may opt to take either estrogen-replacement therapy (ERT) or hormone-replacement therapy (estrogen plus progestin, HRT).

This can be a difficult decision. On the plus side, taking hormones usually relieves hot flashes, appears to protect bones, and may lower an older woman's risk of heart attack by reducing her cholesterol level and increasing the amount of HDLs, the "good" cholesterol, that are circulating in her blood. But hormone therapy also has a down side, as it raises the risk of developing breast and uterine cancers. This puts women in the uncomfortable position of protecting their heart and bones at the cost of their breasts and uterus. (Note: Estrogen does not appear to protect the male heart. In fact, an early test in the long-running Framingham, Massachusetts, study that first identified the link between cholesterol and heart disease showed that men given estrogen were more likely than others to develop blood clots, an adverse effect of estrogens. And they were also more likely to develop the heart attacks that estrogen was supposed to prevent.)

The search for a safer therapy has led to the creation of drugs that prevent estrogen from exerting some of its cancer-promoting effects, such as linking up with estrogen receptors in breast tissue. These drugs, sometimes called "anti-estrogens," are also known as "designer" or "targeted" estrogens. The first, tamoxifen (Nolvadex), is being used to treat breast cancer patients. The recent results of the National Cancer Institute's Breast Cancer Prevention Trial suggest that when it is taken by healthy women, it may reduce their chance of ever developing breast cancer. The second, raloxifene (Evista), appears to protect bones and may also reduce a healthy woman's risk of developing breast cancer.

But these drugs are far from perfect. Women who take tamoxifen for more than five years triple their risk of uterine cancer; raloxifene is so new that right now nobody knows whether it is safe for long-term (longer than two years) use. You will read more about designer estrogens in Chapter Four, "Soy, the Cancer Fighter." Right now, let's talk about another alternative to estrogen, the natural estrogens derived from plants.

FABULOUS PHYTOESTROGENS

Because plants and people are outwardly so different, you may be surprised to discover that many different plants, including soybeans, produce natural chemicals that act like estrogen or interact with it. In science-speak, the prefix *phyto* means "plant." Chemicals from plants are called phytochemicals; estrogens from plants are called phytoestrogens.

Folk medicine has a long tradition of using plants with phyto-estrogens as contraceptives or abortifacients (substances that cause miscarriage). For example, the ancient Greek physician Hippocrates knew that eating the wild carrot, later known as Queen Anne's lace, prevented women from becoming pregnant. Modern scientists explain why: Its seeds contain a chemical that inhibits progesterone, the female hormone that enables a fertilized egg to implant firmly in the wall of the uterus.

Scientists, as opposed to folk practitioners, have also known about phytoestrogens for decades. One early article, appropriately if unimaginatively entitled "Estrogen and Related Substances in Plants," appeared more than 40 years ago in the journal *Vitamins and Hormones*. In 1971, the National Academy of Sciences included a very short review of the then-current literature on phytoestrogens in the second edition of *Toxicants Occurring Naturally in Foods*, a classic rogues' gallery of food hazards much beloved by food, chemistry, and nutrition junkies.

These early reports on phytoestrogens centered on their effects, mostly unpleasant, on animals who ate them by accident while for-

Table 2-2 Some Plant Foods Containing Phytoestrogens

Anise	Garlic
Apples	Hops
Carrots	Parsley
Cherries	Pomegranates
Coffee beans	Potatoes
Dates	Rice
Fennel	Soybeans
Wheat	

Sources: National Research Council, *Environmental Estrogens and Other Hormones* (CBR, Tulane, and Xavier Universities, New Orleans); *Toxicants Occurring Naturally in Foods,* Second Edition (Washington, D.C.: National Academy of Sciences, 1973).

aging in open fields. But in 1990, at a workshop sponsored by the National Cancer Institute, a group of scientists identified a series of anticancer agents, including phytoestrogens, in soybeans and soy products. Since then, the nutritional spotlight has turned to the intriguing possibility that phytoestrogens from plant foods such as herbs and spices, potatoes, and soybeans may not only reduce our risk of cancer but may also serve as safe alternatives to natural and synthetic estrogens, offering the benefits of hormones without the risks.

Table 2-2 lists some common plant foods that contain phytoestrogens.

The phytoestrogens in these and other foods divide naturally into several different categories. The three most important are isoflavones (found abundantly in soy), lignans, and coumestans.

Isoflavones

Isoflavones pop up in many different kinds of food, but there's absolutely no doubt that the food with the most abundant amounts are the legumes, particularly soybeans and soy foods.

Isoflavones are almost universally believed to be the substances in soy proteins that produce most of the health benefits attributed to soy foods. According to Kenneth D. Setchell of Children's Hospital

Table 2-3 The Isoflavone Content of Soy Foods

Food	Serving	Isoflavones
Soybeans	½ cup	35 mg
Soy flour	½ cup	50 mg
Tofu	½ cup	40 mg
Tempeh	½ cup	40 mg
Miso	½ cup	40 mg
Soy milk	1 cup	40 mg
Soy sauce	–	0
Soy oil	–	0
Soy protein concentrates	*	*

*Depending on how they were processed, soy protein isolates may or may not contain isoflavones. Generally, soy protein concentrates are not good sources of isoflavones.

Source: United Soybean Board, Soy Facts #7, *Soyfoods and Isoflavones*, (Seattle, Wash.).

and Medical Center in Cincinnati, the amount of isoflavones in the soy proteins commonly used in our foods often reach levels as high as 3 milligrams per gram of soy, making soybeans and soy products the only foods from which we get nutritionally significant amounts of isoflavones. In fact, some studies suggest that as little as 1 cup of soy milk, or ½ cup tofu, gives us a sufficient amount of isoflavones to produce measurable effects in our bodies.

Table 2-3 lists the isoflavone content (in milligrams) of common servings of soy foods.

Daidzin and Genistin

The most important isoflavones in soybeans are genistin and daidzin. Together they comprise more than 95% of all the isoflavones in the bean.*

*Here's a horticultural curiosity: When soybeans are planted seems to influence their isoflavone content. Beans planted late in the growing season, at the end of June rather than in the middle of May, have nearly twice the isoflavone content of beans from early plantings.

Your body cannot absorb daidzin and genistin. Luckily, when you eat soy products, the bacteria in your gastrointestinal tract convert these isoflavones to compounds you can use easily. Genistin becomes genistein; daidzin becomes daidzein.

Both genistein and daidzein have a chemical structure similar to estradiol, the estrogen made in the ovaries of female mammals. Initially daidzein is more easily absorbed than genistein, but once again, your intestinal bacteria accommodate your body. They break genistein apart into chemicals that are also easy to absorb. Then the daidzein and genistein metabolites (break-down products) move from your intestinal tract through the large portal vein to your liver, out into your blood to circulate through your body and eventually be excreted in your urine. This entire process and the bacteria that make it possible are so efficient that the circulating levels of isoflavones in your blood may be equal to the levels of the estrogens you secrete on your own.

The bacteria that digest daidzin also produce a third isoflavone called equol. A diet that is rich in soy foods is strongly associated with higher levels of equol in your body. Exactly how high varies from person to person, depending on individual body chemistry as well as the natural movement of food through your gut. The longer diadzin lingers in your digestive tract, the more equol your bacteria make. If your body moves food slowly along your digestive tract, you make more equol. If you speed food quickly through, you make less.

What Isoflavones Do

In many ways isoflavones behave just like estrogens. Like estrogen molecules, molecules of soy isoflavones attach themselves to estrogen receptors, special sites in hormone-dependent tissues such as breast, ovarian, and uterine tissues (see Chapter Four, "Soy, the Cancer Fighter"). Like estrogen, soy isoflavones appear to lower your total cholesterol levels, thereby reducing your risk of heart disease (see Chapter Three, "Soy and Your Heart"). Like estrogen they preserve bone (see Chapter Five, "Building Better Bones with Soy") and alleviate the intensity of hot flashes (see Chapter Six, "Soy: Hot News About Hot Flashes").

The crucial difference is that daidzein and genistein's estrogenic effects are much weaker than those of either natural or synthetic estrogens. It takes about 100,000 molecules of daidzein or genistein to produce the same effect as one molecule of estradiol. One isoflavone molecule hooking up to an estrogen receptor simply won't have the power of one estrogen molecule hooking up to the same site. "It's like putting the wrong key in a lock," says Mark Messina, a former National Cancer Institute researcher who has studied the estrogenic properties of isoflavones for nearly a decade. "The key might fit, but it won't turn the lock."

Nevertheless, what looks like a weakness is really a benefit in disguise. Like tamoxifen and raloxifene, daidzein and genistein are anti-estrogens. Every molecule of daidzein or genistein that links up to an estrogen receptor displaces a more powerful estrogen molecule that might stimulate the growth of tissue—or tumors. In addition, isoflavones slow down angiogenesis, the creation of the new blood vessels that are required for tumor growth. Finally, unlike natural and synthetic estrogens, isoflavones are not stored in body fat, so their effects on your body are short-lived.

These three characteristics—the ability to displace estrogen molecules, the ability to inhibit tumor growth, and their quick exit from your body—suggest isoflavones as safe substitutes for estrogens. This is an important possibility because isoflavones also seem to have anti-cancer properties. To date, more than 100 studies worldwide have demonstrated that when genistein is added to cells in laboratory dishes or vials, it dramatically inhibits the growth of many different kinds of cancer cells and interrupts the spread of breast, colon, lung, and prostate tumor cells, as well as leukemia cells. In addition, soybeans and soy products contain other chemicals, such as protease inhibitors and antioxidants, that appear to enhance the anti-cancer effects of phytoestrogens. These interactions are described in detail in Chapter Four, "Soy, the Cancer Fighter."

The Other Phytoestrogens

Two other kinds of phytoestrogens in food deserve some mention here. The first, the lignans, are more likely to show up at your dinner table than the second, the coumestans.

Lignans   Plant lignans are phytoestrogens that are most commonly found in grains. Our intestinal bacteria break plant lignans apart to create the "human lignans" enterodiol (END) and enterolactone (ENL), the latter a rearranged version of the former.

Human lignans are weakly estrogenic. Like other isoflavones, they hook up with estrogen receptors in sensitive tissue such as that of the breast. Do they prevent cancer? Right now, the evidence for their cancer prevention in human beings is scanty, and some researchers suggest that the lignans' most important task may be to help us digest the soy isoflavones daidzin and genistin.

Human lignans are eliminated in urine, so one good way to measure the amount of lignans you produce from food is to measure the amounts of lignans you excrete when you urinate. Several clinical studies using this method have found that women on a macrobiotic diet, a regimen consisting almost entirely of grains, excrete much higher amounts of lignans than do women whose diet includes food from animal products.

In 1982, Herman Adlercreutz of the University of Helsinki in Finland found that women excreting small amounts of enterolactone had a higher risk of breast cancer. Fifteen years later David Ingram and his colleagues at the Queen Elizabeth II Medical Centre in Perth, Australia, set up a study to test the Adlercreutz theory. He recruited 144 volunteers, ages 30 to 84, who had just been diagnosed with breast cancer, plus 144 other subjects (who matched the demographic profiles of the cancer patients) to act as controls. Measuring the subjects' urine excretion of lignans over a 72-hour period, Ingram's team found that women who did not have cancer excreted up to 50% more enterolactone than did women with cancer. As a group, the 25% of women excreting the smallest amounts of enterolactone were three times more likely to have breast cancer than were the 25% of women excreting the largest amounts of enterolactone. The women excreting the lowest amounts of equol were four times more likely to have breast cancer. The real question, said Stephen Barnes of the University of Alabama in Birmingham, is whether the lignans are the primary factors in reducing the risk of breast cancer or whether they are a marker for something else.

The grain with the highest amount of lignans is flaxseed. Ounce for ounce, it can deliver as much as 75 to 800 times more lignans than any other plant food. Flaxseed lignans are easily absorbed, and people who eat flaxseed readily excrete lignans in their urine, more so than with other grains. In one study that was underwritten by the Minnesota Association of Wheat Growers, nutrition researcher Joanne L. Slavin fed 28 healthy volunteers, who usually ate very little fiber, two different high-fiber diets. The fiber in the first diet came from flaxseed; in the second one, from wheat bran. On the flaxseed diet, the volunteers excreted significantly increased amounts of lignans; on the wheat bran diet, they did not.

Right now, the most obvious benefit of consuming lignans appears to be that they serve as additional fuel for the bacteria that turn indigestible daidzin and genistin into digestible daidzein and genistein. END and ENL, the "human lignans" these bacteria produce, are water-soluble, weakly estrogenic chemicals. Like other phytoestrogens, they, too, hook up with estrogen receptors in hormone-sensitive body tissues. Only time will tell whether they are actually anti-cancer chemicals, but here's an intriguing clue. As Claire Hasler of the University of Illinois has written on her soy and human health information web page, mammary cancers are rare among our cousins the apes, who normally excrete significant amounts of dietary-derived lignans in their urine.

By the way, the fact that phytoestrogens, including lignans, are excreted in urine has allowed us to see that men and women use phytoestrogens differently. The amount of phytoestrogen by-products a man excretes is "dose dependent." The more he takes in, the more he eliminates. A woman's body doesn't work that way. Her excretion of phytoestrogen byproducts does not depend on how much she consumes. Exactly what this means is unclear, but it suggests that women may be holding more lignans that are linked to estrogen-sensitive tissue.

Coumestans   The third, and—in human dietary terms—least important group of phytoestrogens are the coumestans. The best-known coumestan is coumestrol, an estrogenic compound found primarily in alfalfa (there are also insignificant amounts in soybeans and soybean sprouts).

Coumestrol has stronger estrogenic effects than the isoflavones. It is more likely than genistein to stimulate the growth of uterine tissue in immature mice, and, unlike the isoflavones, it is stored in body fat. Consequently, it is no surprise to learn that coumestrol can have deleterious effects, the most common being interference with reproduction.

Cattle and other grazing animals who consume alfalfa with high levels of coumestrol often become infertile, while birds and mice who eat coumestrol-laden grains produce fewer offspring. In laboratory studies, rat pups exposed to high doses of coumestrol in their mother's milk have suffered permanent reproductive damage. As adults, the females did not ovulate and the males had difficulty ejaculating.

Coumestrol is most dangerous when the foods containing it make up the bulk of an animal's diet. Therefore, coumestrol does not threaten our reproductive health. Yet we would be foolish not to note its effects on animals and equally foolish not to ask this question: If phytoestrogens act like estrogens and if estrogens may be hazardous for some women, can we simply take it for granted that the phytoestrogens we get from food are safe?

THE SAFETY OF PHYTOESTROGENS

Perhaps the most logical way to begin talking about the safety of phytoestrogens is to explain how plants themselves use these chemicals. Like all living things, plants need to protect themselves against predators—in this case, animals that eat plants. From the plant's point of view, phytoestrogens such as coumestrol are an effective weapon in a classic defense strategy, sacrificing the current generation to save future ones. When sheep or cattle or other grazing animals forage on plants high in coumestrol or eat corn infected with fungus that encourages production of yet another phytoestrogen, zearalenone, they become infertile. A smaller number of lambs or calves are born, and the threat to the plants left standing is reduced.* Clearly, phytoestrogens may be hazardous for animals. But what about human beings?

*Plants are not the only estrogenic reproductive hazards animals face. There are similar accounts of reproductive damage to animals that were exposed to synthetic chemicals, such as pesticides that have estrogenic effects. For example, Louis J. Guillette, Jr., of the Department of Zoology at the University of Florida in Gainesville, has written about alligators in Florida's Lake Apopka that have been exposed to these estrogenic pollutants. Frequently, their eggs do not hatch, or their offspring hatch but do not survive, or the ones that do survive have undeveloped reproductive organs.

Individual Differences

As Roger A. Clemens, a nutrition scientist with the Nestle Company, told the audience at the Institute of Food Techologists' annual meeting in June 1997, a slew of individual variables, most prominently age, affect isoflavones' behavior in the human body.

Early in a woman's reproductive life, when her body is bursting with natural estrogens, isoflavones are likely to be protective. Weakly estrogenic daidzein and genistein molecules displace stronger estrogen molecules on hormone sensitive tissue, reducing the risk of estrogen-triggered breast cancer and cancer of the uterus. Perhaps that is why Asian women living in Asia have a naturally lower incidence of these tumors than do women born in the United States or Asian women who emigrate to this country and begin to eat less soy. But after menopause, when the natural secretion of estrogens declines, will phytoestrogens be equally protective—or might they turn out to be a dangerous stimulant?

Infants may face a different risk. In 1995 and 1996, a group of New Zealand researchers began to question the safety of the high levels of phytoestrogens in soy milk formulas for infants. "Some phytoestrogens act as an anti-hormone to the naturally occurring estradiol, inhibiting its activity," they wrote. "This may be beneficial to adults, but for infants it can be deleterious because estradiol is essential to the imprinting and development of many physical, physiological, and behavioral characteristics during the neonatal period and infancy."

As of this writing, there is no hard evidence to show that soy formulas actually harm an infant's body, but the New Zealanders point to the animal studies showing that rats exposed to phytoestrogens in utero develop reproductive problems later in life. And they stress the cautionary tale of another estrogenic chemical, diethylstilbestrol (DES). DES was prescribed for pregnant women for more than 20 years before doctors discovered that reproductive cancers were appearing in girls who were born to women who had taken the drug while pregnant. Given that experience, the New Zealand Department of Health suggests that it would be foolish to ignore the possibility of developmental problems associated with certain phytoestrogens, a concern that is seconded by our own Food and Drug Administration.

The New Zealanders recommended that routine sales of soy formulas be stopped, and that parents use soy formulas only on the advice of a doctor.

Food versus Supplements

In 1954, Martin Stob, the author of the chapter on phytoestrogens in *Toxicants Occurring Naturally in Foods,* wrote that we are unlikely to suffer ill effects from phytoestrogen-bearing plants either "because the plants containing the compounds do not constitute a significant portion of the diet or because the quality of estrogenic compounds is too low to exert physiological effect."

This is still considered an accurate assessment. Phytoestrogens are very weak estrogens, and, unlike the estrogens we take in products such as birth control pills or hormone-replacement therapy, isoflavones and lignans from common foods are not stored in our body fat, so they influence us for short periods of time. As long as we consume them in moderation, from food, they do not appear to be hazardous to healthy adults.

But phytoestrogens do behave like hormones, so it makes sense to think that if you consume very large amounts of them you may run into trouble. That's one good reason to get your phytoestrogens from food rather than from supplements. A second good reason is that right now, nobody really knows exactly what constitutes an "effective" dose of phytoestrogens. And even if we did know, it would be difficult to get what we need from the supplements that are currently on the market. Unlike drugs, dietary supplements—including those containing soy proteins and their isoflavones—are rarely available in standardized doses, which means that it's virtually impossible for you to tell precisely what quantities of phytoestrogens you are getting from brand to brand or even from batch to batch. On the other hand, if you want to know the phytoestrogen content of your soy food, all you have to do is turn back to Table 2-4.

For the time being, play it safe and stick to soy foods. That way, you not only get reasonable amounts of phytoestrogens, you also get vitamins plus minerals plus fiber plus protein plus other valuable chemicals, such as the bone-building omega-3 fatty acids you'll read more about in Chapter Five, "Building Better Bones with Soy."

A Final Word on Soybean Safety

Remember Yu Xi-ong and Gong Gangshi, those intrepid Chinese wanderers who discovered the soybean? Remember, too, that they were probably also the first people to cook the soybean and thus disarm the chemicals in the raw beans that can inactivate several vital enzymes in the human body—a good example for all of us to follow.

SUMMING UP

Like the hormones we make in our own bodies, the hormone-like chemicals in plants influence our tissues and organs. Unlike our own hormones, though, phytoestrogens may offer the benefits of hormones without the risks we have come to take for granted.

In the slightly less than 10 years since the National Cancer Institute workshop turned up its list of anti-carcinogenic phytochemicals, nutritionists have been working furiously to unravel the mysteries of phytoestrogens, including soy's isoflavones, diadzin and genistin. Along the way, they have begun to understand the mechanisms by which the mild and mundane soybean not only fights cancer but also improves digestion, alleviates some of the natural discomfort of growing older, and protects the organ at the very center of the body, the muscular pump whose 100,000 daily contractions provide the oxygen that powers our every action and thought. It is that story to which we now turn.

3

Soy and Your Heart

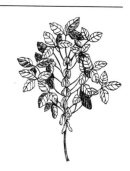

HEART DISEASE AND ITS VICTIMS

The Merck Manual is a medical textbook found in virtually every American doctor's office and on every medical writer's bookshelf. It lists nearly three dozen different kinds of diseases affecting the heart, with descriptions of everything from arrhythmia (an irregular heartbeat) to cancer. But when you and I talk about "heart disease," what we really mean is coronary artery disease, the steady buildup of fatty deposits that narrow and may eventually block a major blood vessel, stopping the flow of blood through the heart—in other words, a "heart attack."

According to the American Heart Association, more than 13 million Americans have some form of heart disease. As many as 1.1 million suffer a heart attack each year, and about one-third of them will not survive. Before the age of 60, a man's risk of heart disease is much greater than a woman's. For example, Table 3-1 shows that among men and women ages 29 to 44, the incidence of heart attack is nearly four times higher among men than among women.

But as Americans grow older, the picture changes. After menopause, when a woman's natural secretion of estrogen declines, her cholesterol levels go up, her HDLs go down, and her risk of heart attack spirals upward. At this point, a woman's risk of heart attack is nearly equal to a man's. Worse yet, American Heart Association statistics show that women who suffer a heart attack are less likely than men to survive. Women who have heart attacks are more likely

Table 3-1 Number of Americans Estimated to Suffer a Heart Attack Each Year

Age	Gender	Number of Heart Attack Victims
29–44 years	male	32,000
	female	9,000
45–64 years	male	218,000
	female	74,000
65+ years	male	418,000
	female	356,000

Source: American Heart Association, *Heart & Stroke Facts*, 1998 Statistical Update.

than men to die within a few weeks; 44% of women who have a heart attack die within a year compared to only 29% of the men. Within six years after a first heart attack, 31% of the women will have a second one, compared to only 23% of the men.

While there is certainly a possibility that a woman's body reacts more violently to the trauma of a heart attack, many experts suggest that a more likely explanation for the lower survival rate among women is that a woman's symptoms of heart disease are not taken as seriously as a man's, which means that women are sicker by the time they get treatment.

Risk Factors for Heart Disease

Epidemiologists attempt to predict who's at risk of heart disease by toting up a person's risk factors, the conditions that make it more likely your body will develop coronary artery disease. The risk factors for heart disease generally fall into one of three categories. First are the risk factors you can't control, such as being male or having a family history of heart disease. Second are the risk factors you can control, such as smoking. Third is the in-between category of risk factors, such as high blood pressure, high cholesterol levels, and diabetes, for which you may have a genetic predisposition but whose effects you can ameliorate. For example, many people gain weight as they grow older, increasing their risk of Type II, non-insulin-dependent diabetes, which consequently increases their risk of heart disease. Controlling your weight lowers your risk of diabetes and high blood pressure, which in turn . . . well, you get the picture.

Table 3-2 lists the risk factors for coronary artery disease, as compiled by the National Cholesterol Education Project.

In the spring of 1988, the American Heart Association added a new risk factor to the list: high blood levels of triglycerides. Chemically speaking, triglycerides are substances composed of one unit of glycerol and three units of fatty acids. In dietary terms, triglycerides are the primary fat in food. You use the triglycerides you get from food to make body fat and lipoproteins, the fat-and-protein particles that carry cholesterol through your bloodstream. And when you need energy, enzymes in your fat cells break up triglycerides so you can burn them for power.

The Heart Association's announcement about triglycerides is based on the results of an eight-year study of 2,906 Danish men, middle-aged and older. When they entered the study, none of the men had any signs of heart disease. Over the years, however, many began to develop heart disease and some had heart attacks. This happened most often among men with the highest levels of "fasting

Table 3-2 Risk Factors for Coronary Artery Disease

Gender	male
Age	over 45 for men
	over 55 for women
Family history	heart attack or sudden death in father or brother younger than 55 or mother or sister younger than 65
High blood pressure	treated or untreated
Diabetes	treated or untreated
Low HDL cholesterol	below 35 mg/dL
Smoking	current

Source: Lawrence M. Tierney, et al., ed. *Current Medical Diagnosis and Treatment*, 37th Ed. (Stamford, Conn.: Appleton & Lange, 1998).

triglycerides" (triglyceride levels in blood samples taken after the men had fasted for 12 hours).

As you can see in Table 3-3, triglyceride levels lower than 200 mg/dL are commonly considered safe. But in the Danish study, the risk of heart disease and heart attack began to rise when triglyceride levels were as low as 142 mg/dL.

It's important to remember that having one or more of the risk factors for heart disease doesn't necessarily mean that you will have a heart attack. While it is better not to have these risk factors or to ameliorate their effects whenever possible, they are simply ways of determining the odds, not of predicting actual disease.

CHOLESTEROL AND YOUR HEART

Of all the risk factors with which you have to contend, the one that gets the most attention is cholesterol. Cholesterol is an important constituent of your body's tissues. It keeps cell membranes healthy, enables you to send messages back and forth between nerve cells, and makes it possible for your body to synthesize hormones, vitamin D, and digestive bile acids.

That's the good news. The bad news, as you certainly know, is that cholesterol is carried on lipoproteins, some of which pass through blood vessel walls and ferry the cholesterol into the arteries. There, it latches onto microscopic tears in the vessel wall, snaring passing cells to form fat-and-cell deposits, called plaques, that

Table 3-3 Triglycerides: What's Normal?

<200 mg/dL	normal
200–400 mg/dL	borderline high
400–1,000 mg/dL	high
>1,000 mg/dL	very high

Source: American Heart Association, "Study Suggests Triglyceride Levels May Be Considered an Independent Risk Factor for Heart Attack in Some People" (March 23, 1998).

may ultimately narrow the artery and block the flow of blood, causing a heart attack.

Measuring Cholesterol

One way to estimate how much cholesterol is circulating in your blood, though not necessarily how much cholesterol is glomming up your arteries, is the cholesterol blood test, which measures the number of milligrams of cholesterol in one deciliter (tenth of a liter) of blood. On your annual health report, the results look like this: 225mg/dL. Translation: You have 225 milligrams of cholesterol in every tenth of a liter of blood.

As a general rule, if your cholesterol level is above 250 mg/dL, you are said to be at "high risk" for heart disease. If your cholesterol level is between 200–250 mg/dL, you are at "moderate risk." A cholesterol level below 200 mg/dL means you're at "low risk." According to the American Heart Association, after age 50, women generally have higher cholesterol levels than men do. At ages 50 to 59, 35% of white females and 36% of black females have cholesterol levels at or higher than 240 mg/dL, but only 32% of white males and 24% of black males are in the same range. After age 60, the number of women with cholesterol levels at or above 240 mg/dL rises to 41% compared to only 26% of white men and 30% of black men.

What Cholesterol Levels Mean

It's important to point out that risks based on total cholesterol readings are only guidelines and your total cholesterol level may be a less important predictor of heart disease than your level of protective HDLs. According to Robert B. Baron, M.D., and Warren S. Browner, of the University of California at San Francisco, this is especially true for women. Therefore, one simple way to estimate your risk of heart disease using both your total cholesterol level and your HDL level is to calculate your cholesterol/HDL ratio (your total cholesterol divided by your HDLs).

Here's how it works. Say your total cholesterol level is 248 and your HDL level is 51. To get your ratio, you divide 248 (the total cholesterol) by 51 (the HDL cholesterol) and get a ratio of 4.9. This number represents a point on a scale that was created through a study funded by the National Health, Lung, and Blood Institute and was based on information obtained from participating lipid (fat) research clinics throughout the United States. The scale predicts heart attack risk for men ages 40 to 44, but the same number may imply a higher risk for people who are younger than 40 or a lower risk for people older than 44. Therefore, when you have a blood test, a computer at the laboratory that does the test will indicate the risk implied by your own ratio at your age. For example, a 60-year-old man with an cholesterol/HDL ratio of 4.9 would be at a lower risk than a younger man with the same ratio.

Table 3-4 shows the risk implied by various cholesterol/HDL ratios for men and women ages 40 to 44.

Cholesterol/HDL ratios are easy to do and easy to understand. But here's a caveat. The American Heart Association says that they're not as accurate a diagnostic or predictive tool as your HDL, LDL, and triglyceride levels. We still go with serum lipid levels, says Mary Winsten, senior scientist at the American Heart Association headquarters in Dallas.

So what's the best real-life advice? Read all the numbers, check your family tree, cut back on risk factors you can control—then relax. Preferably, as you are about to find out, with a soy burger in hand.

Table 3-4 Risk Ratios for Coronary Heart Disease for Men and Women Ages 40 to 44

Risk	Men	Women
Lowest	less than 3.8	less than 2.9
Low	3.9–4.7	3.0–3.6
Moderate	4.8–5.9	3.7–4.6
High	6.0–6.9	4.7–5.6
Highest	more than 7	more than 5.7

*These levels are for people ages 40 to 44. If you are older or younger, the laboratory that evaluates your blood test will automatically adjust the figures to reflect your age.

Source: Lipid Research Clinic.

SOY VERSUS CHOLESTEROL

In many parts of the world where soy is an important part of the diet, the incidence of coronary artery disease is lower than in the United States. For example, in 1991, there were approximately 238 deaths from cardiovascular disease for every 100,000 men in Japan versus 487 deaths for every 100,000 men in the United States. For Japanese women, the number of deaths per 100,000 is 121 versus 232 in the United States. In China, the risk of heart attack is lower for men, but not for women.*

These encouraging statistics are no accidents. More than 40 years of animal and human studies show that eating soy lowers cholesterol, reduces the incidence of blood clots, helps to control weight, protects against high blood pressure, and—most recently—lowers homocysteine levels, too.

Early Hints

In 1967, nutrition scientists produced the first tentative evidence of soy's ability to protect the health of the heart. In a small study, with only 30 volunteers, all of whom had moderately elevated cholesterol levels, those who agreed to try a diet using texturized soy protein foods instead of animal protein foods experienced at least a 20% reduction in their cholesterol levels.

Since that small but encouraging trial, there have been more than 40 studies with men and women, older people and young ones. Every time, when the researchers added up the numbers at the end of the study, the conclusion was exactly the same: Substituting soy protein foods for some or all of the animal protein foods in your diet lowers your cholesterol.

For those who like their figures neat, I am delighted to be able to tell you that the results of 38 major studies on the effects of soy on your heart are summed up in a 1995 meta-analysis (a study of many other studies) by James Anderson of the Metabolic Research Group at

* In France, where practically no one substitutes soy protein for animal protein and lots of people eat high-fat foods, the incidence of cardiovascular disease is also lower than in the United States. The usual explanation for this phenomenon, known as the French Paradox, is the higher consumption of wine.

the Veterans Administration Medical Center and the University of Kentucky in Lexington.

The Anderson Meta-Analysis

The Anderson meta-analysis covers 38 studies with more than 730 volunteers. Thirty-four of the studies were limited to adults; four also included children. In each study, volunteers substituted soy protein foods for protein foods from animals: mixing isolated soy protein into other foods; using texturized soy protein products in place of meat, fish, poultry, and eggs; or drinking liquid formula diets with exactly the same nutritional content except for the protein source, which was either soy foods or casein (the protein in milk).

Some studies compared the soy diet to a "typical" Western diet. Others compared it to a classic low-fat/low-cholesterol regimen (less than 30% of the calories from fat: 300 mg or less of cholesterol a day). The amount of protein provided by the experimental diets ranged from 17 to 124 grams a day; the average was 47 grams a day.

The results? Regardless of who the volunteers were, which diet the soy was paired with, or how much soy protein the regimen provided, the results were exactly the same.

- Eating soy protein instead of animal proteins led to an average 9.3% decline in total cholesterol.
- On soy diets, HDL levels rose 2.4%, which is not considered statistically significant but is considered highly unusual because in most cholesterol-lowering programs, HDLs go down along with total cholesterol.
- On soy diets, LDL levels dropped an average of 12.3%. In nine studies, volunteers experienced a small decrease in LDLs (up to 15 mg/dL). In nine studies, volunteers experienced a moderate decrease in LDLs (20 to 40 mg/dL). In seven studies, volunteers experienced a large drop in LDLs (60 to 110 mg/dL). In two studies, there was a small (5 to 10 mg/dL) increase in LDLs; in five studies, there was no change; six studies did not report LDL results.
- The people who scored the steepest decline in cholesterol and LDL levels on soy diets were those whose original readings were in the

"high" 250 to 289 mg/dL range. People with high cholesterol levels experienced a drop of 24%; for those who started the study at lower, "normal" levels, cholesterol levels went down about 7.7%; in other words, the higher your cholesterol is to begin with, the better your response to soy is likely to be.

Table 3-5 shows the results of the 39 studies included in the Anderson meta-analysis.

SOY'S CHOLESTEROL BUSTERS

The Anderson meta-analysis gave researchers an answer to this basic question about soy and diet: Do people who benefit from a diet that substitutes soy protein for animal protein do better because they're eating soy or because they're on a vegetarian diet?

It's definitely the soy, says Belinda Smith, a nutrition researcher working with Dr. Anderson. She explains that people who start a vegetarian diet usually lose weight and lower their cholesterol levels simply because a vegetarian diet is lower in fat, which means lower in calories and lower in cholesterol.

But the studies in the Anderson meta-analysis compared soy diets with low-fat, low-cholesterol diets providing precisely the same nutritional content. The volunteers on the soy diets and those on the control diets were getting exactly the same amount of calories, fat, saturated fat, and cholesterol (the cholesterol in the soy diet came from protein-free animal fat). Yet in the end, there was a significant difference. Cholesterol levels fell further among people who got their protein from soy rather than from animal products. (Note: According to Elzbieta M. Kurowska of the University of Western Ontario, Canada, whole soybeans have a stronger effect on LDL/HDL ratios than other forms of soy food, such as oil alone or soy protein alone.)

"We don't know for sure what the active ingredient in soy is," said Belinda Smith, "but we expect it may well be the isoflavones." This assumption that the credit goes to estrogenic isoflavones is entirely logical because it's practically a medical truism that natural and synthetic estrogens lower the overall cholesterol and LDLs, while raising HDLs. That's why a woman's risk of heart attack is almost always lower than a man's prior to menopause and why so

Table 3-5 The Anderson Meta-Analysis: 38 Studies of Soy's Effects on Cholesterol Levels

Date Results Published	Journal (Author*)	Number of Subjects (Gender)	Amount of soy per day ISP/TSP+	Fat/ cholesterol Levels@	Effect on LDL Cholesterol&
1977	Lancet (Sirtori)	20 (m/f)	47 g TSP	N/A	moderate decrease
1978	Federal Pro. (Carroll)	6 (f)	47 g ISP/TSP	similar (fat) less (chol)	N/A
1978	Federal Pro. (Carroll)	10 (f)	44 g ISP/TSP	similar	N/A
1980	Lancet (Descovich)	27 (m/f)	47 g TSP	similar	large decrease
1980	Atherosclerosis (Holmes)	12 (m/f)	27 g TSP	similar	no change
1980	Atherosclerosis (Holmes)	10 (m/f)	62 g TSP	similar	no change
1981	American Journal of Clinical Nutrition (Shorey)	24 (m)	51 g ISP	similar	N/A
1981	Journal Reports Int. (Wolfe)	7 (m)	47 g ISP	N/A	large decrease
1981	American Journal of Clinical Nutrition (van Raaij)	24 (N/A)	54 g ISP	similar	moderate decrease
1982	American Journal of Clinical Nutrition (van Raaij)	20 (N/A)	53 g ISP	similar	small decrease
1982	American Journal of Clinical Nutrition (van Raaij)	20 (N/A)	55 g ISP	similar	small increase

Date Results Published	Journal (Author*)	Number of Subjects (Gender)	Amount of soy per day ISP/TSP+	Fat/ cholesterol Levels@	Effect on LDL Cholesterol&
1982	Atherosclerosis (Fumagalli)	4 (m/f)	39 g ISP	similar	N/A
1982	Atherosclerosis (Fumagalli)	3 (m/f)	39 g ISP	similar	N/A
1982	Atherosclerosis (Goldberg)	12 (m/f)	90 g ISP	similar	small decrease
1982	Atherosclerosis (Goldberg)	4 (m/f)	90 g ISP	similar	small increase
1982	Human Nutri. Applied Nutr. (Vessby)	6 (m/f)	37 g TSP	similar (fat) less (chol)	moderate decrease
1983	Journal of Lipid Research (Sacks)	13 (m/f)	27 g ISP	similar (fat) N/A (chol)	no change
1984	Am. Journal of Clinical Nutrition (Huff)	5 (m)	41 g ISP/ TSP	similar (fat) higher (chol)	moderate decrease
1985	Annals Nutri. Metab. (Sirtori)	65 (m/f)	47 g TSP	similar (fat) less (chol)	moderate decrease
1985	Annals Nutri. Metab. (Sirtori)	65 (m/f)	23 g TSP	similar (fat) less (chol)	N/A
1985	Atherosclerosis (Verrillo)	19 (m/f)	31 g TSP	similar	large decrease
1985	Atherosclerosis (Verrillo)	38 (m/f)	31 g TSP	similar (fat) less (chol)	large decrease
1986	Nutrition Res. (Giovanetti)	12 (f)	71 g ISP	similar	small decrease
1986	Transmondial (Widhalm)	11 (m/f) $	20 g ISP	N/A	moderate decrease
1987	Am. Journal of Clinical Nutrition (Gaddi)	16 (m/f) $	56 g TSP	N/A	moderate decrease

(continued on next page)

Table 3-5 The Anderson Meta-Analysis: 38 Studies of Soy's Effects on Cholesterol Levels *(continued)*

Date Results Published	Journal (Author*)	Number of Subjects (Gender)	Amount of soy per day ISP/TSP+	Fat/ cholesterol Levels@	Effect on LDL Cholesterol&
1987	Am. Journal of Clinical Nutrition (Gaddi)	20 (m/f)	75 g TSP	similar (fat) less (chol)	large decrease
1987	Nutrition Rep. Int. (Mercer)	5 (m/f)	17 g ISP	similar	no change
1987	Journal of Clinical Invest. (Lovati)	12 (m/f)	64 g TSP	similar	large decrease
1988	Atherosclerosis (Meinertz)	10 (m/f)	113 g ISP	similar (fat) higher (chol)	no change
1988	Atherosclerosis (Meinertz)	11 (N/A)	124 g ISP	similar	no change
1989	Atherosclerosis (Jenkins)	11 (f)	28 g ISP	similar (fat) less (chol)	small decrease
1991	Am. Journal of Clinical Nutrition (Laurin)	9 (m/f) $	31 g ISP	N/A	small decrease
1992	Australian Journal Nutrition Diet. (Steele)	14 (m/f)	21 g ISP	N/A	moderate decrease
1992	Australian Journal Nutrition Diet. (Steele)	18 (m/f)	26 g ISP	N/A	moderate decrease
1993	American Journal Nutri. Diet. (Potter)	25 (m)	50 g ISP	similar	moderate decrease
1993	Journal of Pediatrics (Widhalm)	23 (m/f) $	18 g ISP	N/A	moderate decrease

Date Results Published	Journal (Author*)	Number of Subjects (Gender)	Amount of soy per day ISP/TSP+	Fat/ cholesterol Levels@	Effect on LDL Cholesterol&
1994	Journal of Nutrition (Bakhit)	21 (m)	25 g ISP	similar	small decrease
1994	Journal of Nutrition (Bakhit)	11	25 g ISP	similar	small decrease

* Author indicates the name of the researcher who wrote the article in which this study appears. This author may be reporting his or her own study or comparing the results of studies done by other persons.

+ ISP = isolated soy protein; TSP = texturized soy protein.

@ Indicates whether the soy diet was similar, higher, or lower in fat and cholesterol than the control diet.

$ Study included children.

& This number represents the mean; some people experienced a higher or lower decline in LDLs.

Source: Anderson, James. W., et al., "Meta-Analysis of the Effects of Soy Protein Intake on Serum Lipids," *New England Journal of Medicine* (August 3, 1995).

many physicians recommend hormone-replacement therapy after menopause begins.*

*Because taking estrogen at menopause increases the risk of endometrial cancer, many physicians recommend estrogen plus progestin for women who have not had a hysterectomy. But does this combination also protect the heart? In April 1998, the American Heart Association journal *Circulation* carried the results of a three-year, 100-woman study in the Department of Cardiology at Skejby University Hospital, Aarhus, Denmark, suggesting the answer may be "No." Taking estrogen enables a woman's blood vessels to expand more easily, thus reducing her risk of heart attack. In the Danish study, the women were divided into two groups, one given an estrogen/progestin combination and the other, no therapy. At the end of the trial, there was no apparent difference between the groups. Unlike estrogen alone, the combination did not make vessels more flexible. According to cardiologist Robert Vogel, this "raises a red flag that progestins may undo some of the cardiovascular benefits of" estrogen replacement therapy.

Isoflavones and Your Heart

Many animal studies show that phytoestrogens do the same thing. For example, when laboratory monkeys are given soy proteins that are high in isoflavones, their fat and cholesterol levels go down, whereas animals that are given soy proteins from which the phytoestrogens have been extracted show only minimal effects.

Based on the evidence of his own meta-analysis, James Anderson estimated that soy's phytoestrogens may account for 60% to 70% of the cholesterol-lowering effects of soy proteins in human beings. Cesare R. Sirtori, director of the Center E. Grossi Paoletti at the Institute of Pharmacological Sciences of the University of Milano, disagrees with the estimate of the importance of isoflavones and adds three additional reasons why soy products may be important to heart health: fiber, protein, and antioxidants.

Soy Fiber and Heart Health

Everyone who is familiar with modern nutrition knows that the soluble fiber in beans, including the soybean, reduces the amounts of cholesterol circulating in your blood. One theory is that the soluble gums and pectins in beans dissolve in the liquid in your stomach, forming a gel that binds with cholesterol and moves it out of your body. A second possibility is that the soluble fiber serves as food for the bacteria in your colon, which digest it to produce chemicals called long-chain fatty acids. These, in turn, suppress your liver's natural production of cholesterol. Beans also contain insoluble fiber, the lignin, hemi-cellulose, and cellulose in the bean's "skin." Insoluble dietary fiber prevents constipation by moving food quickly through your intestinal tract, and this, too, may lower the amount of cholesterol you absorb from food.

Soy Proteins and Your Heart

Like soy fiber, soy proteins seem to speed your body's excretion of cholesterol. One theory is that soy proteins bind with steroid chemicals such as cholesterol and move them quickly to the lower part of the intestine so that they are eliminated in feces. This appears to be what happened in a study run by a team of Japanese and Chinese nutrition researchers from the University of Ryakyus and the University of Occupational and Environmental Health Hospital in Japan, Providence University (Taiwan), and the Fuji (Japan) Oil Company.

For one month, young women volunteers were given a diet whose protein came from either casein or soy. The women who got soy protein excreted higher amounts of steroids (remember, cholesterol is a steroid chemical). In addition, their HDLs rose and their LDLs fell, always a gratifying result in cholesterol research. William W. Wong, of Baylor College of Medicine in Texas, theorizes that soy's ability to step up excretion of cholesterol is what makes substituting soy foods for animal protein foods so effective in tandem with the classic low-fat, low-cholesterol diet.

Cesare Sirtori has suggested a second way in which soy proteins may lower cholesterol levels. The cholesterol you get from food is processed by your liver, and then sent out on lipoproteins into your bloodstream. In addition, your liver churns out about 1 gram (1,000 mg) of cholesterol a day, regardless of how much cholesterol you get from food. Looking for a way to explain why people who substitute soy protein for animal protein end up with cholesterol levels 20% to 24% lower than when they started, the Sirtori team zeroed in on the soy protein itself. What they found was that substituting soy foods for animal protein in an animal's diet causes "significant increases" in activity in the animal's liver at receptor sites that catch and hold LDLs. The researchers have called for more detailed studies to find out whether this also happens in human beings and whether it explains why people who eat soy can lower their own production of cholesterol.

Soy Antioxidants and Your Heart

Finally, all fruits and vegetables, including the soybean, contain antioxidant chemicals such as the tocopherols (vitamin E) and ascorbic acid (vitamin C), which prevent molecular fragments called free radicals from hooking up with other molecules or fragments of molecules that injure your tissues. Tocopherols travel through your bloodstream attached to lipoproteins. The tocopherols traveling on LDLs may prevent these "bad" cholesterol particles from damaging artery walls.

Soy's antioxidants also seem to protect against cholesterol damage. When agricultural researcher Mary Astuti of Gadjah Mada University in Bulaksumur, Indonesia, gave laboratory rats either the fermented soy product tempeh, plain soybeans, or casein (the protein in milk), she found a marked drop in cholesterol and triglyceride levels in the blood of rats who got either tempeh or soy. The best results occurred among rats given tempeh, which appeared to work by reducing levels of malonaldehyde (MDA), an enzyme the rats need to process fats such as cholesterol.

Adding Soy to an Anti-Cholesterol Diet

Because there is no cholesterol in plant foods, the simplest way to cut back on dietary cholesterol is to eat more grains, fruits, vegetables, nuts, and seeds. Foods from animals do contain cholesterol, but you can reduce the amount of cholesterol you get from meat, fish, poultry, eggs, and dairy foods by restricting your daily consumption of these foods to portions that enable you to keep your total cholesterol intake below 300 mg.

Table 3-6 lists the amount of cholesterol in representative servings of common foods from animals.

A second way to lower your cholesterol is to control the amount of fat and saturated fat in your diet. A diet high in fats, particularly saturated fats, is likely to raise the amount of fat (including cholesterol) in your blood. Monunsaturated and polyunsaturated fats do not appear to raise cholesterol. In fact, they may actually reduce the amount of fat circulating in your blood. Vegetables and vegetable oils, including soybeans, soy foods, and soybean oil, are high in polyunsaturated and monounsaturated fats.

How Much Soy Protects Your Heart?

The data from the 38 studies included in the Anderson meta-analysis show that adding as little as 25 grams of soy protein to your diet each day can reduce your total cholesterol level by an average of 8.9 mg/dL. Doubling the soy doubles the reduction: 50 grams of soy a day may produce a 17 mg/dL drop in total cholesterol.

Table 3-7 shows the average drop in serum cholesterol levels among people consuming three different amounts of soy protein a day.

Table 3-6 The Amount of Cholesterol in Representative Servings of Common Foods from Animals

Food	Serving	Cholesterol (mg)
Meat		
beef, stewed, lean	2.2 oz	66
beef, ground, lean	3 oz	74
beef steak, sirloin	3 oz	77
bacon	2 strips	11
pork chop, lean	2.5 oz	71
Poultry		
chicken, roast		
white meat	3 oz	73
dark meat	1.6 oz	41
turkey, roast		
white meat	3 oz	59
Fish		
clams	3 oz	43
flounder	3 oz	59
oysters	1 cup (raw)	120
salmon		
canned	3 oz	34
baked	3 oz	60
tuna		
canned, spring water	3 oz	48
Dairy products		
butter	pat	11
cheese		
American	1 oz	27
Cheddar	1 oz	30
cream	1 oz	31
mozzarella		
whole milk	1 oz	22
part skim	1 oz	15
Swiss	1 oz	26
Eggs		
yolk, large	1	213
white, large	1	0
Milk		
whole	8 oz	33
1%	8 oz	18
skim	8 oz	10

Source: USDA, *Composition of Foods*, USDA Handbook #8-16 (Washington, D.C., 1988).

Table 3-7 Decreases in Serum Cholesterol Linked to Soy Proteins

Amount of Soy Protein	Average Decrease in Cholesterol
25 g/day	8.9 mg/dL
50 g/day	17.4 mg/dL
75 g/day	26.3 mg/dL

Source: Anderson, James W., et al., "Meta-Analysis of the Effects of Soy Protein Intake on Serum Cholesterol," *New England Journal of Medicine* (August 3, 1995).

According to the American Heart Association, every 1% reduction in your serum cholesterol level decreases your risk of heart attack by 2% to 3%. Given the results detailed in the Anderson meta-analysis, adding a few servings of soy foods to your normal diet might actually lower your risk of coronary artery disease 18% to 78%—which kind of makes you wonder why the American Heart Association has not endorsed the health benefits of plain soy.

As you can see from Table 3-8, which shows the soy protein content of common servings of soy foods, adding 25 grams of soy protein to your normal diet is a cinch. At breakfast, you can divide 1 cup of soy milk (7 grams of soy protein) between your cereal and

Table 3-8 Soy Protein Content of Various Soy Foods

Soy Food	Amount	Soy Proteins (grams)
Soybeans		
cooked	½ cup	14
roasted	½ cup	34
Soy flour	¼ cup	8
Soy milk	1 cup	7
Tempeh	½ cup	16
Texturized soy protein	4 ounces	11
Tofu	4 ounces	10

Source: United Soybean Board, Soy Facts #5, *Soyfoods & Heart Disease* (n.d.).

your coffee or tea. At lunch, serve up 4 ounces of stir-fried tofu (10 grams of soy protein). At dinner, toss ½ cup of cooked soybeans on your salad (14 grams of soy protein). Tote up the numbers and, bingo! you've got 31 grams of soy protein, more than 20% over your mark.

Obviously, there are other ways to fit soy protein into your daily menu. You can mix texturized soy protein into meatballs, substitute soy burgers for beef burgers, serve up a no-cholesterol frozen tofu dessert, or simply snack on soy nuts. Any choice you make will benefit your heart.

BEYOND CHOLESTEROL

Lowering cholesterol is not soy's only gift to your heart. Modern research shows that this wonderful bean may also prevent blood clots, lower homocysteine levels, and help you control your weight and your blood pressure.

Preventing Blood Clots

You bleed when a blood vessel wall is torn. To prevent blood loss, tiny particles called platelets flow to the site, forming a plug in the blood vessel wall. When a large blood vessel is injured, the walls of the vessel contract, attempting to hold back the flow until platelets arrive to create a plug. At the same time, chemical changes caused by the injury activate proteins called coagulation factors, which coalesce into strands of fibrin, a substance that builds a strong protein network in the platelet plug.*

Ordinarily, blood clotting is a life-saving mechanism. But when a blood clot forms in a narrowed vessel, it may block all blood flow resulting in a heart attack or stroke. To dissolve current clots or prevent future ones, heart attack victims are given heparin or aspirin, anti-coagulant "blood thinners" that keep platelets from clumping

---

*People with bleeding disorders, such as the various forms of hemophilia, lack specific coagulating factors necessary to create the platelet plug and keep blood from flowing out of their blood vessels. For them, every injury holds the prospect of serious blood loss or painful bleeding into joints.

together or interfere with the formation of protein based clots. But what, you may ask, has that to do with soy? The answer is that the isoflavone genistein seems to act like a mild anti-coagulant.

Blood clotting is triggered by molecules called reactive oxygen species (ROS) that are produced when platelets are stimulated. In laboratory experiments, adding genistein to blood samples from rats slows down the enzyme-related changes in platelets that lead to blood clots. The more genistein is added to the test tube, the lower the production of clots.

In other laboratory studies, researchers have found that adding genistein to a test tube containing platelets and smooth muscle cells not only prevents the platelets from clumping, but also slows the growth of the smooth muscle cells. This is a very significant discovery. Your blood vessels are lined with smooth muscle. When the muscle is damaged, fat and cholesterol particles may be snagged at the site of the injury, creating a "net" that catches smooth muscle cells flaking naturally from the artery wall as well as other cholesterol particles floating by. The resulting pile of cholesterol particles and smooth muscle cells forms a plaque. As it enlarges, it may eventually block the artery, causing a heart attack. If genistein behaves in your blood vessels as it does in the test tube, it might help prevent the plaque from forming in the first place.

Reducing Homocysteine Levels

For the last three decades, Americans have wrestled with what might be called the Cholesterol Contradiction: Some people with high cholesterol live practically forever, yet others with desirable cholesterol levels die young.

As you know, one way to explain this anomaly is to say that it isn't just the total cholesterol level that counts. The HDLs and LDLs are also important. High levels of low-density lipoproteins (LDLs) are bad; high levels of high-density lipoproteins (HDLs) are good (one benefit of the new anti-cholesterol drugs, called "statins," is that they lower total cholesterol and LDL levels while increasing the levels of HDLs).

Now there's a second explanation for the Cholesterol Contradiction: homocysteine. Homocysteine is an amino acid that is released when your body digests proteins. High blood levels of homocysteine appear to increase your risk of heart attack by damaging the smooth muscle cells in the lining of your arteries, by promoting their growth (which could lead to arterial blockage), or by triggering blood clots. As a result, many heart researchers have come to believe that high levels of homocysteine may be an independent risk factor for heart disease, perhaps as important as your cholesterol level.

Luckily, soy foods may play an important role in lowering homocysteine levels. First, soy has less homocysteine than animal foods, so substituting soy products for animal foods immediately lowers the amount of homocysteine in your blood. Second, soy is high in B vitamins. In 1997, while checking through the records of more than 80,000 women who were enrolled in the long-running Nurses Health Study, Eric B. Rimm, M.D., of the Harvard School of Public Health, found the first direct link between two B vitamins and heart health. Rimm's discovery is that a diet providing more than 400 mg of folate (folic acid) and 3 mg of vitamin B_6, either from food or from supplements, may cut a woman's risk of heart attack practically in half by lowering the amount of homocysteine circulating in her blood. For the record, 3.5 ounces of tempeh gives you 52 mg folate and 0.3 mg vitamin B_6, 13% and 10%, respectively, of the protective doses. It's not much, but every little bit counts.

Weight, Blood Pressure, and Your Kidneys

Soybeans can help you win the battle of the bulge, reducing the potential damage from another important risk to your heart: high blood pressure. As we age, many of us tend to gain weight. This can be especially troublesome for women at menopause. In 1998, an analysis of data from the Nurses Health Study showed that women who gain more than 22 pounds after age 18 are twice as likely to have high blood pressure as women who stay within four pounds of their weight as an 18-year-old. The good news is that losing weight and keeping it off lowers blood pressure, particularly in women who are already overweight or who are younger than 45. Women who are overweight at 18 and lose at least 22 pounds as they grow older lower their risk of high blood pressure by as much as 25%.

High blood pressure makes your heart work harder to pump blood out into your body. This may damage the artery walls, reducing their ability to expand and to carry sufficient blood and oxygen to your organs. The result is an increased risk of heart disease, stroke, and kidney disease.

American Heart Association statistics show that one of every four adult Americans has high blood pressure. But there are no symptoms. The only way to find out if you are among that 25% is to be tested. To do that, your doctor wraps a rubber cuff attached to a gauge called a sphygmomanometer around your upper arm and inflates the cuff, compressing a large artery in your arm. This temporarily restricts the flow of blood. Then, listening through a stethoscope pressed against an artery in the crook of your elbow, he notes the pressure registered on the gauge at the moment when your heart beats, sending blood into your arteries, and then when it relaxes between beats.

Your blood pressure is written as two numbers, such as 130/80. The first, higher number is the systolic pressure, the force exerted against artery walls when your heart beats. The second, lower number is the diastolic pressure, the force exerted between beats. What's high blood pressure? Repeated readings at or higher than 140/90.

As a low-fat, high-fiber food, soybeans obviously belong in any diet designed to lower your weight, which will also help to control your blood pressure.

Another way that soybeans control your blood pressure is by reducing your risk of kidney disease. Your kidneys eliminate the nitrogenous waste material produced when you digest and metabolize proteins. As you grow older, even if your kidneys are completely healthy, they begin to work more slowly. Eating lots of animal protein, which is high in fat and cholesterol, may accelerate this natural decline because digesting animal protein produces relatively large amounts of nitrogenous waste material, which makes the kidneys work harder. In this case, the end result may be high blood pressure.

It looks as if soy proteins are more kidney-friendly than animal proteins. In one study with rats that had part of their kidneys removed, Maria Gabriella Gentile and Guiseppe D'Amico, of the San Carlo Borromec Hospital in Milan, found that a diet with protein derived solely from vegetables and soybeans reduced damage to kidney tissue, lowered the amount of protein excreted in urine by 38%, reduced cholesterol levels by 28%, and lowered LDL cholesterol by 33%. "We suggest that the vegan soy diet may have considerable benefit in patients with kidney disease and that lowering serum cholesterol levels may protect the kidneys as well," said Gentile and D'Amico.

A second study lends weight to this conclusion. The subjects were eight men who had non-insulin-dependent diabetes, a condition with complications that include kidney disease. After eight weeks on a standard diabetes diet, the men were divided into two groups: the first group received protein from soy (soy beverage and meat alternatives); the second, from animal foods (milk and beef). At the end of the trial, the men on the soy diet had better kidney function. The researchers theorize that the soy isoflavones genistein and equol behave like the diuretic drug furosemide (LASIX), preventing the body from reabsorbing salt, which can stress the kidneys (for more on these and other chemicals in soybeans, see Chapter Two, "Something Special in the Bean").

And Don't Forget . . .

Even if this is a book about soybeans, no one can end a chapter on heart health without adding a few words about smoking and physical inactivity, two important risk factors for heart disease.

Smoking is first on everyone's list of lifestyle problems that are linked to heart disease. Tobacco contains nicotine, a vasoconstrictor that narrows blood vessels. Whenever you inhale nicotine in tobacco smoke or absorb it into your bloodstream by sniffing snuff or chewing tobacco, your blood vessels constrict, which is why you feel a slight, pleasurable rush whenever you puff. Unfortunately, the rush also signals a brief increased risk of heart attack due to narrowed blood vessels.

Better to get your rush from physical activity. Lying around like a couch potato promotes obesity, which raises cholesterol levels and blood pressure. Working out, running, or just plain walking briskly for 40 minutes three or four times a week helps to control your weight. Losing weight will help to lower your blood pressure and your total cholesterol level, while raising your levels of protective

HDLs—the "good" fat and protein particles that carry cholesterol and fats out of your arteries and out of your body.

Listen, being fit doesn't require that you look like a Bay Watch babe or a bodyguard. It just requires your getting up and moving around. Is there an easier way in the world to look good, feel good, and be kind to your heart?

SUMMING UP

Along the way to arriving at a serious scientific conclusion, there is a really great moment when things suddenly reach what might be called critical mass.

All of the studies are pointing in the same direction. The evidence is reasonable. The conclusions seem valid for human beings as well as animals. And you get this wonderful feeling that you are about to be able to say something valuable about how to make people healthier.

That's where we are right now with soy and your heart. It's clear that substituting soy protein for protein from animal foods lowers cholesterol levels, improves the ratio of protective HDLs to destructive LDLs, prevents excessive stress on the kidneys, helps control weight, and consequently helps control blood pressure. Exactly how soy performs this magic remains to be proven, but there is no longer any doubt that the versatile soybean—high in fiber and with no cholesterol, a favorable ratio of unsaturated fatty acids, and all those wonderful phytoestrogens—belongs in every heart-healthy kitchen.

4

Soy, the Cancer Fighter

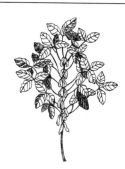

THE STATISTICS OF CANCER

Every year, the American Cancer Society publishes a list of the ten most common cancers in the United States and the ten leading causes of cancer deaths. The most recent ACS statistics are listed on the following charts.

Table 4-1 shows the number of estimated new cases of the most common cancers among men in 1998, the last year for which figures are available. Table 4-2 shows the most common cancers among women. Table 4-3 shows the leading causes of cancer deaths among men. Table 4-4 shows the leading causes of cancer deaths among women.

Table 4-1 Estimated New Cases of the 10 Most Common Cancers Among Men in the United States/1998

1.	Prostate	184,500
2.	Lung	91,400
3.	Colon and rectum	64,600
4.	Bladder	39,500
5.	Non-Hodgkins lymphoma	31,100
6.	Melanoma (skin)	24,300
7.	Oral	20,600
8.	Kidney	17,600
9.	Leukemia	16,100
10.	Stomach	14,300

Source: American Cancer Society, Cancer Facts and Figures—1998.

Table 4-2 Estimated New Cases of the 10 Most Common Cancers Among Women in the United States/1998

1. Breast	178,700
2. Lung	80,100
3. Colon and rectum	67,000
4. Uterus (endometrium)	36,100
5. Ovary	25,400
6. Non-Hodgkins lymphoma	24,300
7. Melanoma (skin)	17,300
8. Bladder	14,900
9. Pancreas	14,900
10. Cervix	13,700

Source: American Cancer Society, Cancer Facts and Figures—1998.

Run your finger down these lists, and you will see that the leading cancers among men and women in the United States and the number two causes of cancer deaths are reproductive cancers, cancer of the breast, and cancer of the prostate. Three additional reproductive cancers—cancer of the uterus (endometrial cancer and cancer of the cervix) and ovarian cancer—are also among the ten most common female cancers.

Table 4-3 Estimates of Cancer Deaths Among Men in the United States/1998

Site	Number of Deaths
1. Lung	93,100
2. Prostate	39,200
3. Colon and rectum	27,900
4. Pancreas	14,000
5. Non-Hodgkins lymphoma	13,000
6. Leukemia	12,000
7. Esophagus	9,100
8. Bladder	8,400
9. Stomach	8,100
10. Liver	7,900

Source: American Cancer Society, Cancer Facts and Figures—1998.

Table 4-4 Estimated Cancer Deaths Among Women in the
United States/1998

Site	Number of Deaths
1. Lung	67,000
2. Breast	43,500
3. Colon and rectum	28,600
4. Pancreas	14,900
5. Ovary	14,500
6. Non-Hodgkins lymphoma	11,900
7. Leukemia	9,600
8. Uterus (endometrium)	6,300
9. Brain	6,000
10. Stomach	5,600

Source: American Cancer Society, Cancer Facts and Figures—1998.

These five cancers have three things in common. First, each one is hormone-related. Exposure to estrogen raises the risk of breast cancer, cancer of the ovary, and cancer of the uterus. Exposure to testosterone raises the risk of prostate cancer.

Second, each one is influenced by diet. Healthy, well-fed people produce lots of hormones, reach puberty earlier, have longer reproductive lives, and consequently have a higher risk of hormone-related cancers.

Third, each one is more common today than in the past. In 1960, an American woman's lifetime risk of breast cancer was 1 in 14, and there were about 73 cases of breast cancer a year for every 100,000 women in the United States. Today, the lifetime risk of breast cancer for women who live longer than 85 is 1 in 8, and the incidence of breast cancer has risen to 108 cases for every 100,000 women. There is a similar but more complex rise in the incidence of prostate cancer. In 1940, there were approximately 14 cases of prostate cancer diagnosed among every 100,000 American men. By 1990, there were about 26 cases per 100,000. The first explanation for this nearly 86% increase in the number of cases of prostate cancer is simply that there are many more men living into their 70s and beyond, which is an age when prostate cancer is much more common. The second explanation is that the increase in detection is due to the introduction and use of a simple screening blood test. However, the fact remains that the number of prostate cancer deaths among American men has risen 25%. By 1997, it was the most common cancer among American men, and the American Cancer Society forecast an estimated 41,800 deaths a year, just about 2,000 fewer than the annual number of breast cancer deaths among women—although women who die of breast cancer tend to die at a much earlier age than men who die of prostate cancer.

We have come to accept these terrible numbers as a fact of life in the United States. But what we take for granted may not be true in the rest of the world, and simply changing our Western diet may actually reduce our risk of some kinds of cancer.

Let's start by examining the evidence for diet's effects on cancer risk. Then we'll move on to show that the risk of reproductive cancers is lower among Asians and Asian-Americans than among Americans of other ethnicities, and we will consider whether the Asian experience may hold the key to our own protection against the rising toll of reproductive cancers.

DIET AND HORMONE-RELATED CANCERS

If you believe that what you eat influences your risk of cancer, the odds are that sometime in your life someone called you a "health nut." No longer. Today, constructing a diet that lowers your risk of cancer is definitely mainstream medicine—and it's getting more so every day.

In 1981, British cancer researcher Richard Peto, head of the cancer research unit at Oxford University, estimated that, based on a series of studies linking cancer to specific foods, primarily foods from animals, between 10% and 70% of all cancers might be linked to diet. By 1997, the American Cancer Society had concluded that as many as one-third of the 560,000 cancer deaths that year might be caused by diet, most particularly the high-fat, low-fiber diet that is known to increase the risk of cancer of the colon and rectum, which is the third leading cause of cancer deaths among American men and women.

Study after study points to one clear culprit at the dinner table: fats. A high-calorie diet and excessive amounts of alcohol are also problematic. That's the bad news. The good news is that nutrition experts have also zeroed in on one group of highly protective foods: plants. Particularly the soybean.

Problem Foods

A high-fat diet may increase your risk of cancer in two ways. First, digesting and metabolizing fats produces free radicals, the molecular fragments that combine with other fragments to make potentially carcinogenic molecules. Second, fats are high in calories. They contribute to weight gain, and extra body fat can increase your natural production of sex hormones.

The cancer that is most firmly linked to dietary fat is colon cancer, but the trail from fat to tumor is twisty. The epidemiological evidence seems indisputable: People who eat lots of fats and very little fiber are more likely to develop cancer of the colon. What's confusing is trying to figure out which kind of fat is to blame. In one famously contradictory study of information from the long-running Nurses Health Study, a high-fat diet was firmly linked to an increased risk of colon cancer, but the risk was tied only to fats from red meat: beef, lamb, and pork. Consuming dairy fat had absolutely no effect on a woman's chance of developing colon cancer.

Because some studies show that obesity is a risk factor for breast cancer and cancer of the uterus, and other studies suggest that obesity shortens the survival time for breast cancer patients, it might seem logical to say that a high-fat diet is also a risk factor for breast cancer. But no one has yet established a direct link between the diet and the disease.

What we do know for sure is how to define a high-fat diet. The USDA/Health and Human Services Dietary Guidelines for Americans recommend holding your fat intake to no more than 30% of your total calories. In real-life terms, that means no more than 600 calories a day from fat in a typical 2,000-calorie-a-day diet.

If you consume fewer calories, you should cut your fat intake accordingly. Anything that exceeds the 30% figure can fairly be considered "high fat."

High-calorie diets can also be troublesome. The more calories you take in, the more likely you are to gain weight, which increases your chance of being overweight, which increases your risk of getting certain kinds of cancer, notably cancer of the colon and rectum. Keeping your calories (which means total food intake) in line helps keep your weight within a normal range and protects against these cancers.

Finally, let's talk about alcoholic beverages. Moderate drinking (one drink a day for a woman, two for a man) appears to lower the risk of heart disease, but exceeding these limits can be hazardous to your health. The American Cancer Society estimates that excessive use of alcohol, often in tandem with tobacco, may be implicated in as many as 19,000 deaths a year from oral cancers (mouth, tongue, and throat). For women, even moderate drinking may increase their risk of breast cancer. Some researchers believe that this is due to alcohol's ability to increase the amount of estrogen circulating in a woman's blood; others blame the increased risk of breast cancer on additional life-style choices.

By the way, here's an interesting story about soy isoflavones and alcohol that you can use as cocktail conversation. A Chinese folk remedy for hangover is extract of *Pueraria lobata*, an edible vine that contains three important isoflavones: puerarin, daidzin, and daidzein. In laboratory experiments, rats that were given alcohol through a tube inserted directly into their stomachs were less likely to become intoxicated (which, for rats, means falling into an alcohol-induced sleep) when pueraria extract was mixed in with the alcohol. In addition, among animals who got alcohol plus pueraria, alcohol absorption peaked earlier and blood alcohol levels did not rise as high as they did among animals given alcohol alone.

Giving the animals daidzein by mouth appeared to slow the rate at which alcohol moves from the stomach to the small intestine, where it is absorbed into the bloodstream. It also seemed to suppress the desire for alcohol. Rats fed puerarin, daidzin, and daidzein voluntarily consumed less alcohol and more water, resuming normal alcohol consumption when the isoflavones were eliminated from their feed. Soy canapés, anyone?

Good Guys at the Table

When it comes to fighting cancer, plant foods are your friends, as valuable for this as they are for reducing your risk of heart disease. In the 60 years since a group of British researchers first posited a link between a vegetable-rich diet and a lower risk of cancer throughout the human body, more than 200 epidemiological studies have investigated the anti-cancer role of plant foods. The clear majority of these studies show that people who eat a diet rich in plant foods—not just one kind of vegetable, but all kinds—are much less likely to develop cancer.

As John D. Potter, of the Fred Hutchinson Cancer Research Center and University in Seattle, Washington, explains, plants are virtually bursting with anti-cancer chemicals that interrupt the growth of malignant cells at every stage in the carcinogenic process, from the moment of the original exposure to a cancer-causing agent through changes that allow a cell with abnormal DNA to grow and multiply into a detectable tumor and then to metastasize to other sites.

Antioxidants such as ascorbic acid (vitamin C); the tocopherols (vitamin E); flavonoids*; red, yellow, and orange carotenoid pigments; and the phenols in wine, fruits, and vegetables prevent free radicals from joining other molecular fragments to form carcinogens such as the nitrosamines. Dietary fiber moves food quickly through your body, reducing the formation of potentially carcinogenic compounds, and the bacterial digestion of dietary fiber in your gut produces fatty acids that trigger cell death in cancer cells. The sulfur compounds—glucosinolates, indoles, isothiocyanates, and thiocyanates—that lend flavor and odor to cruciferous vegetables such as cabbage, cauliflower, broccoli, and brussels sprouts stimulate your body's production of enzymes that inactivate carcinogens, inhibiting the growth and multiplication of cancer cells. Phytoestrogens in soy and other plant foods hook up with estrogen receptors in sensitive areas such as the breast tissue, replacing natural estrogens and reducing the risk of hormone-related cancers.

For all these reasons, the suggestion by the Dietary Guidelines for Americans that you have at least 5 servings of fruits and

---

*Animal studies suggest that flavonoids protect the integrity of capillaries, the very small blood vessels just under the surface of your skin, but there's no such evidence that this protective capacity also exists in regard to human beings.

Table 4-5 Anti-Cancer Chemicals in Plant Foods

The Chemical	What It Is/Does
Ascorbic acid	vitamin C, antioxidant
Carotenoids	antioxidant pigments
Dietary fiber	indigestible material in plant foods
Flavonoids	antioxidant pigments
Folate	vitamin that may inhibit the transformation of healthy cells into malignant cells
Glucosinolates*	natural sulfur flavor and aroma compounds
Indoles	a building block for biochemicals formed in the digestion of the amino acid tryptophan
Isothiocyanate*	natural sulfur flavor and aroma compounds
Phenols	antioxidants named for their chemical structure (atoms arranged in rings, rather than straight lines)
Phytoestrogens	natural plant chemicals that act like weak estrogens
Thiocyanates*	natural sulfur flavor and aroma compounds
Tocopherols	vitamin E, antioxidants

*These sulfur-based chemicals create the distinctive aroma and flavor of cruciferous vegetables.

Source: Committee on Food Protection, *Toxicants Occurring Naturally in Food* (Washington, D.C.: National Academy of Sciences, 1973); Mayo Clinic Health Letter, September 1995.

vegetables a day, plus 20 to 30 grams of fiber, makes nutritional and medical sense. (How much fiber is there in a serving? Count on about 4 grams in ½ cup serving of most plant foods, more in beans and peas.)

Table 4-5 lists the anti-cancer chemicals found in common plant foods.

Diet and Breast Cancer

In the last decade, as cancer researchers have built the case for the link between your diet and your risk of cancer, the evidence regarding breast cancer and diet has seemed inconclusive and often confusing. But some diet guidelines have finally begun to emerge in the fight against breast cancer.

You can find a good summary of these findings in the results from the DIANA ("diet and androgens") project at the National Tumor Institute in Milan, a study involving 104 healthy postmenopausal Italian women ages 50 to 65 with a relatively new marker for breast cancer: high-serum testosterone.

As the National Women's Health Network wrote in its Network News health letter in the winter of 1998, several studies among American women (white, African-American, and Latina) have demonstrated that higher ratios of testosterone to estrogen are also linked to higher blood pressure, insulin resistance (the necessity to secrete more insulin than normal to digest food), and higher concentrations of LDLs, the "bad" lipoproteins that carry cholesterol into your arteries.

The DIANA project is the first study designed solely to alter testosterone's effects on breast cancer risk. To reduce testosterone levels, the researchers proposed a diet composed of foods that would reduce insulin levels and lower hormone production. The list includes unrefined cereals and beans; foods with a low glycemic index (meaning your body can digest them with a minimum amount of insulin, thus lowering the natural secretion of other hormones triggered by insulin); nutrients such as omega-3 fatty acids, dietary fiber, vitamin B_6, and chromium, which make insulin more effective so you require less of it to digest your food; foods that are low in animal fats (except for omega-3 fatty acids) to control weight and reduce the accumulation of body fat that is associated with higher blood levels of sex hormones; and foods that are rich in phytoestrogens, to modify the metabolism of sex hormones.

Table 4-6 lists the important chemicals in the foods used in the DIANA project diet and their proposed effects on your body.

Half the DIANA volunteers were randomly assigned to continue their normal diet; the other half were given a diet that conformed to the testosterone-insulin-lowering principals listed in Table 4-6. At the end, the results were undeniable. Cholesterol levels, weight, and testosterone levels dropped among the women on the "anti–breast cancer" diet, confirming the direction in which dietary recommendations have been trending. What we now know, the DIANA team

Table 4-6 The Elements of the DIANA Project Anti–Breast Cancer Diet

Substance	Aim
Phytoestrogens	to reduce the carcinogenic actions of sex hormones
Low glycemic index foods	to decrease insulin levels and reduce synthesis of SHBG
Omega-3 fatty acids, dietary fiber, vitamin B_6	to enhance insulin sensitivity
Less animal fat (except for omega-3 fatty acids)	to reduce body fat associated with higher hormone levels

Source: F. Berrino, "A Randomized Trial to Prevent Hormonal Patterns at High Risk for Breast Cancer: The DIANA (Diet and Androgens) Project," symposium.

wrote, is that if you eat more plants, you can change how your body reacts to the hormonal triggers that ordinarily increase your risk of breast cancer. Now the question is, can this basic anti–breast cancer diet be improved with soy?

THE ASIAN EXPERIENCE

No epidemiologist will deny that hormone-related reproductive cancers are much less common in Asia and in Third World countries than in the United States and the industrialized West. As study after study demonstrates, Asian women seem to have a lower risk of breast cancer than non-Asians do—as long as they remain in Asia. If they emigrate to the United States, their risk rises. For example, in Japan, the annual incidence of breast cancer is 52.3 cases for every 100,000 women. Among women of Japanese descent living in the United States, it is 82.3. For Chinese women, the figures are even more stark. In China, there are 5 cases of breast cancer for every 100,000 women; among women of Chinese descent living in this country, 55.

There is a similar but less well-documented difference among men in the risk of prostate cancer, which is lower in Asia and higher

Table 4-7 Annual Incidence of Breast Cancer in Selected Countries

Country	Cases per 100,000 Women
**United States	108
*Japan	52.3
+Hong Kong	10
+China	5
+Korea	3–4

Sources:
* Pharmaceutical Information Associates Ltd., "Soy Protein May Protect Against Breast Cancer," *Medical Sciences Bulletin* (November 1994), PharmInfoNet Homepage.
**American Cancer Society, Cancer Facts and Figures—1997.
+United Soybean Board, Soy Facts #3, *Soy and Cancer*, n.d.

in the United States. The incidence of prostate cancer among American men of Asian descent, like the incidence of breast cancer among American women of Asian descent, is still lower than the national average.

Table 4-7 shows the annual incidence of breast cancer among women in the United States versus the lower incidence among women living in various Asian countries. Table 4-8 on page 74 shows the incidence of breast cancer among Asian-American women compared to all women in this country.

Why there should be a lower incidence of breast cancer in Asia and why women of Asian descent living in the United States should be less likely than other American women to develop breast cancer are questions that have puzzled researchers for at least two decades.

One possible explanation for the difference in cancer rates is genetics. As you know, Asian women who migrate to the United States and Asian-Americans experience an increase in the incidence of breast cancer, but their risk is still lower than that of other Americans. Perhaps there is something protective in their genetic makeup, say a lower incidence of a "breast cancer gene."

Table 4-8 Incidence of Breast Cancer Among Women of Asian Descent Living in the United States

Ethnic Group	Number of Diagnosed Cases per 100,000 Women
All women in the U.S.*	108
Japanese	82.3
Filipino	73.1
Chinese	55.0
Vietnamese	37.5
Korean	28.5

*Of all races

Source: American Cancer Society, Cancer Facts & Figures—1997.

A second possibility is the fact that estrogen drugs are almost never used in Asian countries. For example, in Japan, the law regarding estrogen prescriptions is so restrictive that practically no one uses either the birth control pill or hormone replacement therapy. As late as 1992, the Japanese Health and Welfare Ministry cited the increasing incidence of AIDS as the reason for keeping in place their long-time restrictions on oral contraceptives, meaning that the condom remains the most widely used method of birth control in Japan.

A third possibility—the one that concerns us here—is diet. Because Asian women living in the United States eat more fat and saturated fat than Asian women living in Asia, some people suggest that the increased consumption of fat raises the risk of breast cancer, but recent studies show no such link. In fact, when it comes to breast cancer, the more significant difference between the Asian and American diets may turn out to be the amount of soy foods each provides.

Soy and Breast Cancer

In 1995, Los Angeles researcher Anna H. Wu and a group of epidemiologists from the National Cancer Institute, the Northern California Cancer Center, and the Cancer Research Center of Hawaii set up a survey that was designed to find out whether the diets of Asian women born in the United States really are different from those of Asian women born abroad.

Armed with a checklist of 90 food items (Do you eat this? What about that?), the epidemiologists questioned 597 breast cancer patients and 966 healthy women. What they discovered was a strong relationship between food choices—specifically soy foods—and the incidence of breast cancer among Chinese, Japanese, and Filipino-American women living in Angeles County, San Francisco, and on the island of Oahu.

After taking age into consideration (older women have a naturally higher risk of breast cancer), Wu concluded that (1) women born in Asia who immigrate to the United States consume about twice as much tofu as Asian-American women born in this country; (2) the longer an Asian immigrant stays here, the less tofu she is likely to eat; and (3) women who eat more tofu are less likely to develop breast cancer.

Tofu's protective effect was evident both in young women and in women who had gone through menopause. It didn't matter what else they ate, simply having tofu in their diet seemed to counteract other risk factors such as early menarche and late menopause. Nevertheless, because the study was not designed specifically to assess the role of soy products, Wu cautions that she "cannot discount the possibility that soy intake is a marker for other protective aspects of the Asian diet and/or Asian lifestyle."

Nevertheless, Wu's study appears to validate the results of more than 20 previous ones, primarily among Asians, showing that even one serving of soy food a day is linked to reduced risk of cancer of the breast, colon, rectum, lung, stomach, and prostate. One good example is the 1994 report published by Mark Messina. Messina's figures show that the number of breast cancer deaths decline as the amount of soy in the diet rises. In Japan, China, Korea, and Hong Kong, where soy consumption is 8 to 30 times higher than in the United States, the number of breast cancer deaths per 100,000 women is as much as 80% lower than in this country.

Table 4-9 shows the correlation between soy consumption and the number of breast cancer deaths in Asia versus the United States.

Table 4-9 Soy Consumption and Breast Cancer Deaths

Country	Average Soy Protein Consumption (grams/day)	Breast Cancer Deaths per 100,000 Women
Japan	30	7
Korea	20	4
Hong Kong	10	9
China	9	8
United States	<1	22.4

Sources: Mark Messina and Virginia Messina, Soy Facts #3, *Soy and Cancer*, United Soybean Board, n.d.

Soy and Endometrial Cancer

In 1997, University of Hawaii researchers interviewed 341 Oahu women of Hawaiian, Japanese, Chinese, Filipino, and Caucasian descent who had been diagnosed with endometrial cancer. The interviewers talked with each woman in her own home, using a standard dietary questionnaire.

Analyzing the answers, the epidemiologists found a strong correlation between a high-calorie diet and a higher risk of endometrial cancer. A high-carbohydrate diet lowered the risk slightly. A high-fiber diet lowered the risk significantly. Overall, the risk of endometrial cancer went down as the consumption of phytoestrogen-rich foods such as beans and peas, whole grains, vegetables, fruit, and seaweed went up. And while all beans and peas were beneficial, the most protective were soybeans. "Our data support the notion that diets low in calories and rich in beans and peas (especially soybeans), whole grain foods, vegetables, and fruits reduce the risk of endometrial cancer," concludes study author Marc T. Goodman.

Soy and Prostate Cancer

The high-soy Asian diet that protects women seems to protect men, too. Like breast cancer among women, prostate cancer is the most common cancer among men and the second leading cause of cancer deaths. And like the incidence of breast cancer among Asian-American women versus women of other ethnic groups, the incidence of prostate cancer is lower among men of Asian descent living in the United States than among American white men or African-Americans.

The differences are remarkable. For every two African-American men with prostate cancer, there is only one man of Japanese descent; for every nine African-Americans, only one Korean-American. For every two American white men with prostate cancer, there is fewer than one Chinese-American; and for every three American white men, only one Vietnamese-American.

Table 4-10 shows the incidence of prostate cancer among American men of Asian descent compared to that of men in other ethnic groups living in the United States.

Soy and Colon Cancer

Unlike reproductive cancers, the incidence of colon cancer among Asian-Americans does not present a simple picture. More than

Table 4-10 Incidence of Prostate Cancer Among Men of Asian Descent vs. Men of Other Ethnic Groups Living in the United States

Ethnic Group	Number of Cases per 100,000 Men
African-American	180.6
White	134.7
Hispanic	89.0
Japanese	88.0
Filipino	69.8
Hawaiian	57.2
Native American	52.5
Chinese	52.1
Vietnamese	40.0
Korean	24.2

Source: American Cancer Society, Cancer Facts & Figures—1998.

100 studies around the world have found that the soy isoflavone genistein inhibits the growth of all kinds of cancer cells—breast, colon, lung, prostate, leukemia—in laboratory dishes. If the isoflavone behaves this way in your body, then the customary Asian diet, with plenty of genistein-rich, high-calcium soy milks and tofus, might explain why the incidence of colon/rectal cancers is lower among Asian-Americans than among other ethnic groups in the United States.

So far, so good. But then you run right smack into a nutritional mystery. Japanese-Americans eat a lot of soy. But, as you can see in Table 4-11, the ethnic group with the highest incidence of colon cancer in this country are Japanese-Americans. Does that mean that soy is not protective? Or is there something unusual in the diet of Japanese-Americans that makes them more susceptible to cancers of the colon and rectum? Right now, nobody knows for sure.

Table 4-11 Incidence of Colon/Rectal Cancer in the United States (by ethnic group)

Ethnic Group	Number of Cases per 100,000	
	Men	Women
Japanese	64.1	39.5
African-American	60.7	45.5
White	56.3	38.3
Chinese	44.8	33.6
Hawaiian	42.4	30.5
Hispanic	38.3	24.7
Filipino	34.4	20.9
Vietnamese	30.5	27.1
Korean	31.7	21.9
Native American	18.6	15.3

Source: American Cancer Society, Cancer Facts & Figures—1997

How Soy Fights Cancer

The soybean is no magic bullet against cancer, but it's hard to imagine another food that gives us more of the phytochemicals that are known to affect the carcinogenic process. Isoflavones, protease inhibitors, and saponins—one at a time or acting in concert, these chemicals may reduce our risk of developing cancer by reducing our exposure to estrogen, countering the effects of testosterone, inhibiting the growth of tumors, and stimulating our immune system.

Soy Reduces Estrogen Exposure

Once your intestinal bacteria convert the soy isoflavones daidzin and genistin into daidzein and genistein (see Chapter Two, "Something Special in the Bean"), these weakly estrogenic molecules begin to link up to estrogen receptor sites in sensitive reproductive tissues, displacing stronger natural and synthetic estrogen molecules and reducing your exposure to their potentially carcinogenic effects.

Soy may also reduce your exposure to estrogen by changing the length of your menstrual cycle, the hormone-mediated event that, as you know, begins with the first day of menstrual bleeding and ends on the last day before the next menstrual bleeding starts. When your cycle starts, your estrogen levels slowly rise and then peak at mid-cycle, when your pituitary gland releases luteinizing hormone (also known as LH or lutropin) to stimulate the release of a mature egg from your ovary. At this point, estrogen levels falls, and progesterone levels rise until menstrual bleeding starts, at which point progesterone levels recede, estrogen levels rise, and the cycle resumes.

The "ideal" female menstrual cycle runs 28 days, but a normal cycle may run longer or shorter. As a general rule, however, Asian women living in Asia have longer menstrual cycles than do American women, including Asian women living in the United States. This is a significant difference. The longer the menstrual cycle, the fewer there will be each year, and the fewer cycles a woman experiences, the lower her exposure to the estrogen that is secreted naturally in her body.

Several recent studies, in which Western volunteers were asked to add soy to their diet or to substitute soy protein foods for protein foods from animals, do show that adding soy to the diet lengthens a woman's natural menstrual cycle. For example, in one small study reported in the November 1994 issue of *Medical Sciences Bulletin*, six healthy women ages 21 to 29 were first given a control diet and then, after a one- to four-month "washout period," a daily diet containing 60 grams of texturized soy protein a day with 45 mg of isoflavones. Blood tests, urine samples, and fecal samples were analyzed to see how fast the soy and isoflavones moved through the volunteers' bodies. The tests showed that the excretion of isoflavones in urine was 1,000 times higher on the soy diet. In addition, two of the women excreted large amounts of equol, the isoflavone that is produced when intestinal bacteria convert daidzin to daidzein.

But here's the part that set the researchers' radar humming. On the high-soy diet, five of the six women experienced menstrual cycles one to five days longer than usual, and the two women who excreted the highest amounts of equol had the longest menstrual cycles. In other words, consuming soy somehow delayed the secretion of the luteinizing hormone, and then that delayed ovulation, a rational explanation for why Asian woman have longer cycles.

Another study of menstrual cycles, this time at the University of Surrey in England, produced similar results. Fifteen healthy volunteers were given a high-soy diet, followed by a control diet with no soy. On the soy diet, their menstrual cycles lengthened, and it took longer for them to reach ovulation. Their cholesterol levels dropped, too, but that's a story you'll find out more about in Chapter Three, "Soy and Your Heart."

By lengthening menstrual cycles, soy foods not only protect the ovaries and uterus, they also protect the breasts. Breast cancer cells divide and multiply much faster at mid-cycle, so lengthening the cycle may also stretch out the time period when the cells do not proliferate, thus reducing the stimulation of breast tumors.*

*Not every study shows that soy lengthens menstrual cycles. At the University of Minnesota, nutrition researcher Mindy Kurzer and a team of obstetricians and gynecologists are investigating the effects of soy isoflavones on premenopausal

Soy Counters Testosterone

At the South Manchester University Hospitals Trust in England, researchers have used soy phytochemicals to slow the growth of human prostate cancer cells in laboratory plates. At Emory University in Atlanta and at the University of Alabama, genistein also appeared to slow prostate tumors that were growing in live laboratory animals.

Rats injected with prostate cancer cells were divided into two groups, one given genistein injections, the others not. Those who got the genistein had smaller tumors that were less likely to invade the surrounding tissue or spread through lymph nodes to other parts of their bodies. And the genistein injections seemed to produce estrogenic effects: PSA* and testosterone levels went down and testes shrank.

Of course, that's a long way from proving that soy will prevent or alleviate human prostate cancers growing in live human beings. What we need is more information from controlled trials such as the one currently in progress at the University of Alabama in Birmingham, where 17 elderly volunteers with higher than normal PSA levels but no current signs of prostate cancer are testing two soy beverages. Both formulas contain 20 grams of isolated soy protein; one also contains genistein. The researchers will track the volunteers' blood levels of PSA, cholesterol, and isoflavones to see if consuming the genistein-enriched drink reduces the risk of prostate cancer.

Soy Slows Tumor Growth

In the spring of 1998, the *New York Times* carried a front-page story describing Harvard researcher Moses Judah Folkman's discovery of

---

women. What makes this study different, Kurzer says, is that "we're not substituting soy proteins for other kinds of proteins. We're measuring the effects of three different amounts of soy phytoestrogens added to the subjects' normal diet. When we look at menstrual cycle data and blood hormone levels, there are almost no changes in the length of menstrual cycles or blood hormone levels, although the difference between this study and others may also be that we're looking at a longer period of time."

*Prostate-specific antigen, a marker for prostate cancer.

endostatin and angiostatin, two drugs that inhibit angiogenesis, the growth of new blood vessels that are required for a tumor to grow and spread. The two drugs have been used successfully in mice, and other drugs that inhibit angiogenesis and shrink tumors have been used in clinical trials with human beings. You're reading about them here because soy's isoflavones also inhibit angiogenesis, another possible explanation for daidzein and genistein's apparent ability to reduce the risk of cancer.

In addition, soy contains protease inhibitors, substances that interrupt the action of enzymes required for cell reproduction and growth. One protease inhibitor in soybeans, known as the Bowman-Birk protease inhibitor (BBI), is so effective at suppressing the growth of cancer cells that it is considered a universal anti-carcinogen.*

In 1986, a group of biologists at the Harvard School of Public Health set up an experiment to examine the effect of protease inhibitors on oral cancer. Painting the inside of hamsters' cheeks with protease inhibitors, the researchers then brushed known carcinogens onto the spots, but no cancers appeared. In a related experiment, adding protease inhibitors to the diet that was fed to laboratory animals protected them from colon cancers.

Soy protease inhibitors may also boost the anti-hormone power of soy isoflavones. At the University of Texas Medical Branch, Galveston, when women volunteers were given 100 mg of daidzein/daidzin, 1,000 mg of genistein/genistin, and 105 mg of protease inhibitors in a 12-ounce soy drink three times a day for one month, their blood levels of estradiol, progesterone, and dehydroepiandrosterone, a weakly androgenic (male) hormone secreted by the adrenal glands, fell 60%, 35%, and 20%, respectively. Among men on the same regimen, blood levels of hormone by-products dropped by as much as 14% after two to four weeks.

Soy Boosts Your Immune System

Beans and peas, particularly the soybean, are a major dietary source of saponins, plant chemicals that foam in water and are capable of

---

*As a class, protease inhibitors' ability to stop replication of the AIDS virus has made them a valuable tool for HIV-positive patients. There is no evidence that soy has any such effect.

injuring cell walls. Recent studies suggest that saponins may lower cholesterol, stimulate the immune system, and counter the effects of carcinogens in your body. Exactly how they do these things remains a mystery, but A. Venker Rao, professor of nutrition at the University of Toronto, says they may behave like antioxidants, preventing the formation of free radicals that damage cells; they may alter the immune system; they may directly attack cancer cells; or they may play a role in regulating cell growth and reproduction. However they accomplish their task, Rao concludes, recent studies in his own laboratory suggest that foods such as the soybean, which are rich in saponins, may be a useful source of natural chemicals that reduce the risk of human cancers.

How Much Soy Should I Eat Each Day?

Studies and reports are fine, but what you really want to know is exactly how much soy you need in your diet to protect yourself against cancer. The best estimates come from studies on breast cancer. In Asian countries where the normal diet commonly contains 9 to 30 grams of soy protein a day, the incidence of breast cancer may be as much as five times lower than in the United States, where we rarely get more than 1 to 3 grams a day (turn back to Table 4-9 for the exact figures). One 1997 meta-analysis of studies on soy consumption and the risk of breast cancer showed beneficial effects at the level of 30 grams a day, the amount in 2 cups of soy milk or 3.5 ounces of tofu, and several studies suggest that as little as 1 serving of tofu a week may significantly reduce your risk.

How much is a serving and what's it worth in terms of soy protein? Table 4-12 on page 84 shows the amount of soy protein in one representative portion of various soy foods.

Should you get your soy protein from supplements? Sorry about this, but as we said in Chapter Two, food is the better way to go. As the North American Menopause Society has posted on its website, dietary supplements such as those promising to deliver soy proteins and/or isoflavones "are rarely 'quality-controlled,' meaning that they have not been tested to make certain each batch is consistent within a manufacturer, or that two different products with the same name have the same components." In addition, "ideal doses of

Table 4-12 The Soy Protein Content of Various Soy Foods

Food	Serving	Soy Protein (grams)
Roasted soybeans	¼ cup	17
Tempeh	½ cup	16
Texturized soy protein	½ cup	11
Tofu	4 ounces	10
Soy flour	¼ cup	8
Soy milk	1 cup	7

Source: "Menopause Online, Soy Foods": info@menopause-online.com.

isoflavones for particular indications have not been well estab-lished," and right now nobody knows if megadose levels of iso-flavones are safe (see the next section).

There's no such problem with soy foods and, like getting your carotene from fruits and vegetables rather than pills, getting your isoflavones from soy foods brings bonuses—vitamins plus minerals plus fiber plus protein plus protease inhibitors plus omega-3 fatty acids. And the food tastes good.

Is Soy Safe?

Because phytoestrogens act like weak hormones, it seems inevitable that very high amounts might have adverse effects. And indeed, in some studies that has turned out to be the case.

Isoflavones and Mice

In 1997, Michigan State University nutrition researcher William G. Helferich found that adding large amounts of genistein to estrogen-dependent and estrogen-independent cancer cells in laboratory dishes made them grow more quickly, at a rate similar to what he would expect to find if he added small amounts of the natural estrogen estradiol.

To see whether genistein would promote or discourage the growth of cancer cells in a living body, Helferich implanted estrogen-dependent cancer cells under the skin of laboratory mice whose ovaries had been removed, meaning that the animals no longer secreted a meaningful amount of natural estrogens. He then divided the mice into three groups. The first group was given estradiol; the second, genistein; and the third (the control group), no hormonal compounds at all. After a short period of time, Helferich measured the size of the tumors in each animal and found that mice who got genistein grew larger tumors than mice who got no hormones. Might that happen to us?

Soy and Human Beings

In evaluating the effects of soy and soy isoflavones on human beings, timing may be everything. Daidzein and genistein exert much weaker estrogenic effects than either natural or synthetic estrogens. Nonetheless, like other estrogens, they bind to estrogen receptors on hormone-dependent tissues. The good news is that in doing this, they displace stronger estrogen molecules. The bad news is that they, too, may stimulate sensitive tissues.

That does not seem to happen when soy is given early on in an animal's life. On the contrary, during one 1995 study cited by University of Illinois soy expert Clare Hasler, rats that were given genistein as newborns were less likely than other rats to develop benign or malignant breast tumors when, at the age of 50 days (middle age for a rat), they were given a chemical known to cause breast tumors. In other words, if given very early in life, soy isoflavones appear to confer an immunity that reduces the animals' long-term risk of contracting breast cancer as they grow older.

Many nutrition researchers think that this may be what happens among Asian women. Because soy is part of their diet from babyhood on, these women are constantly exposed to relatively weak estrogenic substances that bind to breast and other reproductive tissues, displacing the potentially problematic natural estrogens. With so many weak estrogen molecules in place, these lucky women are shielded from the stronger estrogens that may trigger reproductive tumors.

Things might be a bit more dicey for women who are first introduced to soy foods late in life—say, at menopause. "One thing I'm concerned about is that soy may exert some important hormonal effects that may not be beneficial," says University of Minnesota nutrition researcher Mindy S. Kurzer. "We know a lot about women in Asia who have been consuming soy since they were children, but we don't know what it will do to women who start later or how it will affect women with estrogen-dependent cancers."

There are studies showing that eating soy protects bones and relieves some of the signs of menopause such as hot flashes (see Chapter Five, "Building Better Bones with Soy," and Chapter Six, "Hot News About Hot Flashes"), but because older women have naturally low bodily levels of estrogen, it is theoretically possible that the estrogenic isoflavones in soy might act just like hormone-replacement therapy, raising their risk of cancer rather than lowering it.

The data regarding the potentially adverse effects of introducing soy into your diet at menopause is, to put it mildly, incomplete. About the only thing you can say for sure is that you will be hearing more about this one. Meanwhile, it would be smart to bear in mind that the adverse effects of soy isoflavones occur not when animals are given soy foods, but when they are fed (or injected with) high concentrations of isoflavones alone, another argument in favor of food rather than supplements.

A PRACTICAL GUIDE TO YOUR PERSONAL WAR ON CANCER

Despite the advances in cancer research, the causes of many tumors, such as cancers of the pancreas, are still unidentified. As a result, we often feel helpless to protect ourselves. Yet there is much to suggest that we really can reduce the consequences of certain cancers and reduce our risk of succumbing to others by bringing to cancer detection and prevention the same consumer savvy we carry into the rest of our lives.

Early Detection

Cancer is most amenable to cure if we catch it early, before it has spread throughout our bodies. The best way to do this is to schedule regular check-ups. Table 4-13 on page 88 lists common cancer tests for symptom-free people and tells when to take them.

Avoiding Environmental Carcinogens

Americans have known since the 1960s that smoking causes lung cancer. Today we know that cigarette, cigar, and pipe smoke also increases the risk of cancer of the throat and bladder, and maybe cancer of the pancreas and cervix, too. Smokeless tobacco (a.k.a. chewing tobacco) is implicated in cancer of the mouth and tongue.

In 1997, the American Cancer Society warned that there might be as many as 174,000 cancer deaths that year due simply to tobacco use, while another 19,000 deaths could be blamed on smoking plus the excessive use of alcohol or on alcohol abuse alone. Does anyone doubt that the vast majority of these deaths might be prevented if we all stopped smoking and used alcohol in moderation?

A second way to reduce your risk of cancer is to reduce your exposure to environmental carcinogens. Broadly defined, our environment includes our homes, our workplaces, our schools and hospitals, as well as our air and water. Exposure to chemicals and other toxic influences we encounter may clearly affect our risk of getting cancer; this situation was first correctly described in 1775 by an English physician named Percivall Pott, who argued that the high rate of cancer of the scrotum among London's chimney sweeps was due to their constant exposure to soot.

Since Pott's identification of soot as a carcinogen, the list of potential cancer-causing chemicals in our environment has grown to include asbestos, benzene, chloroform, nickel, and vinyl chloride, plus many others. Even those of us who have never set foot inside a chemistry classroom have heard about the potential hazards of PCBs and dioxins. We know that excessive exposure to the rays of the sun may cause skin cancer and that excessive exposure to X-rays, once considered harmless, increases our risk of getting other forms of cancer, including leukemia. We know that natural substances such as aflatoxins (molds that grown on peanuts and other foods) or nitrosamines (chemicals formed in your stomach when you eat foods such as beets, celery, and eggplant) or synthetic chemicals used to produce foods may also be carcinogenic, although their effects depend to a large degree on dosage.

Table 4-13 Scheduling Cancer Tests in People Without Symptoms

Cancer	Test	Gender	Age	Frequency
Colon	Sigmoidoscopy	M & F	50+	Every 1–5 years
	Stool blood test	M & F	50+	Every year
	Digital rectal	M & F	40+	Every year
Prostate	Digital exam	M	50+	Every year
	PSA (blood test)	M	50+	Every year
Cervical	Pap test	F	18+	Every year (after 3 consecutive normal results, at the discretion of the physician)
Ovarian	Pelvic exam	F	18–40	Every 1–3 years, with Pap test
			40+	Every year
Endometrial	Endometrial tissue sample	F	–	At menopause, if high risk; then, at discretion of physician*
Breast	Self-examination	F	20+	Every month
	Clinical exam	F	20–40	Every 3 years
			40+	Every year
	Mammography⁺	F	40–49	Every 1–2 years
			50+	Every year

*"High risk" means a history of infertility, failure to ovulate, abnormal vaginal bleeding, estrogen-replacement therapy (without progesterone), or using tamoxifen.

†In the spring of 1998, a group of researchers led by Joann G. Elmore of the University of Washington School of Medicine and Mary B. Barton of Harvard Medical School and Harvard Pilgrim Health Care (HMO) released the results of a study showing that 24% of 2,400 women who were screened by mammograms had at least one false-positive result (indicating the presence of cancer in a woman who did not have cancer) in a ten-year period. The data suggest that a woman who has a mammogram every year for 10 years after the age of 40 has a 50% chance of getting at least one false positive report in that period. There are 32 million women in this country ages 40 to 70; this rate of error might well add up to 10 million false-positives in any 10-year period.

Source: The American Cancer Society, Cancer Facts & Figures, 1996.

Protecting yourself from carcinogens in the environment is often more difficult than preventing cancer by making a personal decision not to smoke or vowing to eat a diet that is rich in foods known to reduce the risk of cancer. But it is not an impossible task. Today, dozens of chemicals have been banned from your workplace and your home because exposure is known to cause a specific cancer. One good example is benzene—once a popular solvent, now known to cause leukemia. And there have been many new anti-cancer laws, including regulations designed to reduce the risk of medical exposure to radiation from diagnostic machines such as those used to perform mammograms, as well as legislation on both a state and federal level that is designed to reduce our exposure to chemicals from toxic dump sites.

At the same time it is important to deal with real, as opposed to imagined, risks. Because cancer is so common, so often deadly, and still so mysterious, it is a highly emotional subject. So emotional, in fact, that it is often hard to keep fear from conquering reason. Nevertheless, it is to our advantage to make certain that our decisions about cancer prevention are based on sound science.

Most of us worry about four specific kinds of environmental carcinogens: non-ionizing radiation (electromagnetic low-frequency radiation such as radio or electromagnetic waves), pesticides (chemicals used to control insects and weeds), toxic wastes, and nuclear power plants.

While each of these offers reason for legitimate concern—electomagnetic waves may affect enzyme systems in the human body; some pesticides may collect as persistent residues in the tissues of humans and animals; toxic waste dumps do pollute our air, water, and soil; and nuclear power plants do release low levels of ionizing radiation—it is worthwhile remembering that not one of them is as firmly linked to a specific cancer as is the simple, voluntary act of lighting up a cigarette.

Be Cautious with Hormones

Estrogen is a cancer promoter. It stimulates the growth of cells in the ovaries, uterus, and breasts and encourages the proliferation of cancer cells, which is why the known risk factors for breast cancer are a

Table 4-14 Known Risk Factors for Breast Cancer

Family history of breast cancer
Genes (BRCA1/BRCA2) for breast cancer
Early menarche (first menstrual period before age 13)
Late menopause (after age 51)
Recent use of birth control pills
Long-term exposure to postmenopausal hormone therapy
Never having had children
First live birth at a late age
Diet that is high in animal foods
Excessive use of alcohol
Exposure to environmental chemicals (unproven)

Source: American Cancer Society, Cancer Facts and Figures—1997.

veritable catalogue of encounters with estrogen, either the hormone that is produced in your own body or the ones you take as birth control pills and hormone-replacement therapy.

Table 4-14 lists the known risk factors for breast cancer. Caution: This list is not an absolute guide to your own risk of developing breast cancer or other reproductive cancers. True, some women with one or more of these risk factors do develop breast cancer, but others do not. Although we know about the "breast cancer gene," the majority of new cases will still occur in women whose only risk seems to be the fact that they are women, usually older women. As University of Cincinnati radiologist Myron Moskowitz told the National Conference on Breast Cancer in March 1988: "Seventy-five percent of all breast cancers occur in women with no known risk factors."

For men with prostate cancer, the hormone is different but the story stays the same: Testosterone encourages the growth of prostate cancer cells. However, few men use testosterone as medicine, so women are at a higher risk of hormone drug-related tumors.

Thirty-eight years ago, when G. D. Searle introduced the first estrogen/progestin contraceptive pill, an American woman's lifetime risk of breast cancer was 1 in 14. Six years later, when the promotion of hormone- (estrogen) replacement therapy began in earnest with the publication of Robert Wilson's *Feminine Forever*, there were about 73 cases of breast cancer every year for every 100,000 women in the United States.

Today, the lifetime risk of breast cancer for American women who live to 85 is 1 in 8, and the incidence of breast cancer has risen to 108 for every 100,000 women. It would be foolish to attribute the increase in breast cancer cases solely to the use of estrogen drugs, but it would be irresponsible to deny the connection.

Since 1975, more than 12 major epidemiological studies have confirmed a link between the long-term use of birth control pills at an early age and an increased risk of early-onset breast cancer (breast cancer before ages 35 to 40). More than 14 studies confirm a higher incidence of breast cancer among women who are currently using estrogen-replacement therapy or those who use it for long periods of time.*

Today, the connection between hormones and female reproductive cancers is so firmly established that estrogen advocates no longer waste time arguing that estrogen is safe. Instead, they propose the concept of relative risk. Taking estrogen at menopause may raise the risk of breast cancer, they admit, but it lowers the risk of heart disease. Since more women die of heart disease than breast cancer, they say, estrogen is a risk worth taking.

But is that true? Early in the 1970s, it became clear that estrogen-replacement therapy (ERT) could stimulate the proliferation of endometrial cells, which could lead to endometrial cancer. The problem was alleviated by adding progestins to create the estrogen/progestin product called hormone-replacement therapy (HRT). But on May 1, 1997, the American Cancer Society raised a new warning flag when it released the results of a study showing an increased incidence of ovarian cancer among 240,000 postmenopausal women participating in the Cancer Society's 13-year-old prospective mortality study, Cancer Prevention II. According to the ACS, the risk of fatal ovarian cancer was 40% higher for women who used estrogens for

---

*For a comprehensive exploration of the history of estrogen's role in the rising incidence of breast cancer, see Carol Ann Rinzler, *Estrogen and Breast Cancer: A Warning to Women* (Hunter House, 1996).

at least six years and 70% higher at 11 years. Right now, there is no information about whether taking progestins along with the estrogen lowers the risk of ovarian cancer, but as you saw in Chapter Three, "Soy and Your Heart," the estrogen/progestin combination that protects your uterus may not protect your heart as well as estrogen alone.

SUMMING UP

In the past 40 years, dozens of epidemiological studies have shown that people whose customary diet includes a plentiful amount of soy foods are less likely to develop hormone-related cancers of the breast, ovaries, uterus, and prostate.

The credit for soy's ability to prevent cancer goes to its phytochemicals, the isoflavones, protease inhibitors, and saponins that counter the carcinogenic effects of estrogen and testosterone while slowing the growth of tumors and boosting our immune system.

Because isoflavones are estrogenic, there is always the chance that very large amounts may be hazardous. Nevertheless, soy foods have been consumed for centuries; this suggests that the food is safe. If the current trend in scientific studies holds steady, adding soy to our menu may offer us a delicious path to a healthier life.

5

Building Better Bones with Soy

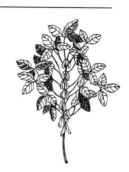

YOUR HORMONES AND YOUR BONES

Like all body tissues, your bones are constantly being replenished. Old tissue is broken down (resorbed) and new tissue is created. The process is initiated by specialized bone cells called osteoclasts, which bore tiny holes into solid bone so that other specialized cells called osteoblasts can refill the open spaces with fresh bone.

This continuing cycle of destruction and renewal is controlled by the sex hormones, estrogen and testosterone, plus a third hormone, human growth hormone (hGH). Estrogen preserves bone by preventing the resorption of excess amounts of bone cells. Testosterone stimulates the growth of stronger, denser bone tissue. Human growth hormone acts as a pilot, directing the pace of new cell production.

Because men always have proportionately more testosterone, the average man almost always has larger, stronger bones than the average woman. Even in early adulthood, when her bones are at peak density, a woman has about one-third less bone mass than a man. As she grows older and her estrogen secretion declines, she conserves less bone tissue and loses more bone density than he does—40% to 50% for women versus 20% to 30% for men.

In the first five years after menopause, a woman may lose as much as 2% of her total bone mass. After that, she is likely to lose about 1% a year for the rest of her life. At the end, she may have lost as much as half of her trabecular bone (the spongy bone in her vertebrae and at the rounded ends of the long bones in her arms and legs) plus 35% of her cortical bone (the denser bone in the middle of the long bones). In the same time period, the average man will lose only 25% of the mass of both his trabecular and his cortical bone combined.

As a result, women are far more likely than men to develop osteoporosis, literally, "bones full of holes." Women are also more likely to suffer bone fractures. Right now in the United States, 15 to 20 million people are living with osteoporosis, and an estimated 1.5 million have suffered a hip fracture, adding about $18 billion in cost to our healthcare system. Of every seven people with a broken hip, six are women.

By far the most important natural mitigating factor against female osteoporosis is the length of your exposure to the natural estrogens produced in a woman's body. In one recent study of white women living in a retirement community in California, Elizabeth Barrett-Connor of the University of California at San Diego, found that nothing (including whether a woman took estrogen) affected bone density, loss of bone tissue, and the risk of osteoporosis more than the total number of her reproductive years prior to menopause. In Barret-Connor's survey, the results were clear: The longer a woman's reproductive life and the more estrogen her body produces, the greater her protection against bone loss as she grows older. In other words, you are less likely to develop osteoporosis if your first period came early (before age 13) and your menopause, late (after age 51).

The best news about osteoporosis, though, is that not every woman is at equal risk. Forget the ads and the promotional hype. Your personal risk of osteoporosis depends on individual factors including, but not limited to, your family history, your own reproductive history, your body type, and your race. For example, if you are small-boned or slim, with very fair skin and very light eyes, and your mother, who looks just like you, broke her hip before age 60, sorry, but your risk of osteoporosis is definitely higher than average.

But black women have a lower-than-average risk of osteoporosis and so do Chinese women living in China. When Chinese women emigrate to the United States, however, their risk rises, perhaps, says Stephanie Atkinson, professor of nutrition in the department of pediatrics at McMaster University in Canada, because "more women are in the labor force in China, with more physical activity that protects against bone loss."

Other aspects of your lifestyle also affect your risk of osteoporosis. A diet rich in calcium is protective. So is the weight-bearing

Table 5-1 Risk Factors for Osteoporosis

Higher Risk	Lower Risk
Family History	
Mother or sister with early menopause	Mother or sister with later menopause
Mother or sister with early fractures	Mother or sister with no early fractures
Reproductive History	
Late menarche	Early menarche
Early menopause	Late menopause
Body Type	
Slim, with small bones, blonde hair, light eyes, fair skin	Large, with large bones dark skin
Race	
Chinese (in U.S.)	Black
Lifestyle	
Smoking	Weight-bearing exercise
	High-calcium diet

exercise because it strengthens bones as well as muscles. Smoking, on the other hand, speeds up bone resorption.

Table 5-1 lists the individual factors that increase or decrease your risk of osteoporosis.

THE HORMONE DILEMMA

Many well-designed studies have shown that estrogen-replacement therapy and estrogen–progestin hormone replacement therapy can play a beneficial role in slowing or even reversing bone loss. But using hormones at menopause raises the risk of getting breast cancer and cancer of the uterus. Some experts say the risk goes up as soon as you start to take estrogen. Others put the danger zone at

7 to 10 years' use. Aiming for a compromise, early in the 1990s many physicians began suggesting short-term (1 to 7 years) hormone-replacement therapy, starting right at menopause when bone is being lost at a fast clip. The idea, of course, was to conserve bone tissue early in the game and then stop using hormones before they could trigger a seriously increased risk of cancer.

It sounds so reasonable, that the news out of the Boston Arthritis Center in 1993 was disturbing to many doctors and their patients. Assessing estrogen use, bone density, and the incidence of bone fractures among 670 Caucasian women in Framingham, Massachusetts, the home of the long-running Framingham Heart Study, the Boston epidemiologists found that women who took estrogen for 7 to 10 years had only about 3% more bone mass than women who never took the hormone, a difference too small to be considered significant. The number of bone fractures among women using estrogen for short periods of time was pretty much the same as the number of fractures among women who never used hormones, although the non-users were likely to have more broken bones in their 60s, which was precisely when most women took estrogen. But the real kicker was that while taking estrogen for less than seven years might temporarily slow the pace of bone loss, it provided no cumulative long-term protection. By age 75, women who had used estrogen short-term showed no more bone density than women who had never used estrogen. In other words, to get lifelong protection against osteoporosis from estrogen, women would have to take hormones for their entire postmenopausal life.

Two years later, an American College of Physicians analysis in the Harvard Women's Health Watch questioned the value of long-term estrogen-replacement therapy, too. According to the ACP report, taking hormones at menopause might reduce a 50-year-old woman's risk of hip fracture by barely 2% to 3%, dropping it from slightly more than 15% to a bit less than 13%. Then, as an aside, ACP noted that because osteoporosis is so rare among African-American women, for them the protective effects of hormones were "insignificant."

While this definitely remains a minority view, it has increased the push for long-term, lower-dose estrogen to protect bones without raising the risk of cancer. In December 1997, scientists at the University of California at San Francisco announced that lower-dose estrogen (0.3 mg/day rather than the usual 0.6 mg/day) halted the loss of bone tissue among 406 postmenopausal volunteers—and, incidentally, reduced their cholesterol levels—with a minimal incidence of such rarely mentioned side effects as the nausea and headache that often lead women to stop taking estrogens. Unfortunately, the UCSF study was too short to see whether lower-dose estrogen comes with a concurrent lower risk of hormone-related cancers.

That is also the problem with raloxifene, a drug approved by the Food and Drug Administration the same week the San Francisco researchers announced their support for lower-dose estrogen.

Raloxifene (Evista) appears to protect bones without an increased risk of breast or uterine cancer. But the backup data on raloxifene submitted to the FDA comes from short-term (two-year) studies among relatively small groups of women. As the National Women's Health Network said in testimony before the FDA panel that approved raloxifene, two years is just not long enough to show whether taking any drugs will increase the risk of breast cancer.

One need look no further for proof than to consider the example of tamoxifen (Nolvadex) to see that the Network is right. Tamoxifen clearly prolongs life by lowering the risk of recurrence among both premenopausal and postmenopausal breast cancer patients when they take it for five years. After that, however, tamoxifen changes its stripes. Women who use the drug for ten years are more likely to suffer a breast cancer recurrence than women who take it for only five years—and they have an increased risk of aggressive endometrial cancer. Note: None of this information denies tamoxifen's value to women with breast cancer. In fact, although the drug was originally prescribed only for women whose cancers were diagnosed after menopause, recent studies show that the prescribed five-year course of treatment may be equally life-saving for younger women. As for raloxifene, it represents an important treatment option for women at high risk of osteoporosis.

In both cases, the question is not whether the drug is useful—clearly, both tamoxifen and raloxifene meet that test—but who should take them? That is, for whom do their benefits outweigh their risks?

Healthy women who do not wish to use hormones or these newer drugs with estrogenic properties need other alternatives.

SOY AND YOUR BONES

Numerous studies over the last two decades have shown that vegetarian women whose diet is high in soy are less likely than other women to develop osteoporosis. And there are always those Chinese women whose bones do better at home, where soy is a dietary staple, than they do here in the United States. Animal studies also attest to soy's protective effects on bone.

The active ingredient appears to be the estrogenic isoflavone genistein. Giving genistein to rats whose ovaries have been removed clearly conserves bone. In one study with 48 rats that were randomized to one of three groups—the first was fed a normal diet; the second, soy protein with isoflavones; and the third, soy protein without isoflavones—Bahram H. Arjmandi of the University of Illinois, Chicago found that the soy-plus-isoflavone diet clearly prevented (but could not reverse) bone loss. Based on this, he advises soy supplementation for menopausal women, and others cautiously agree. "While it is too early to make specific health claims for soy," says the Mayo Health Clinic Health Letter, "there is evidence that adding soy to your diet makes good nutritional sense."*

Genistein performed even better in a study at the University of Kentucky and the Veterans Administration Medical Center in Lexington, Kentucky. Feeding the isoflavone to ovarectomized rats not only conserved bone by suppressing the resorption of old bone cells but actually stimulated the growth of new bone cells. In Lexington, unlike Chicago, the rats who got the genistein held on to the bone they had—and added more.

Among human beings, genistein's benefits to bone have sometimes shown up by accident. In 1996, John W. Erdman, Jr., of the University of Illinois at Champagne Urbana, set up a study designed to see whether eating soy could lower cholesterol levels. Before starting the study, Erdman wanted a base picture of each woman's bones, so he asked each of the 66 postmenopausal volunteers to have dual energy X-ray absorptiometry (DEXA) pictures taken of her whole body, her spine between her ribs and pelvis, and her upper thigh.

The trial began with each woman on a basic low-fat/low-cholesterol diet for two weeks. Next, the volunteers were randomly

---

*Arjmandi's animal studies suggest that the synthetic isoflavone, ipriflavone, also protects against bone loss in rats whose ovaries have been removed.

assigned to one of three diets: (1) the basic diet plus 49 grams of protein from soy protein isolate plus 1.39 mg isoflavones per gram, (2) the basic diet plus 49 grams of protein from soy protein isolate with 2.25 mg isoflavones per gram, or (3) the basic diet plus 49 grams of protein from casein (the protein in milk). To make sure each woman got the same amount of calcium, both soy diets were fortified with calcium equal to that in the casein diet.

When the 26-week study ended, the women had a second set of DEXA pictures. The results were similar to those in the Kentucky rat study. Women on Diet Number Two (soy protein with the most isoflavones) had a significant increase in spinal bone density plus a smaller increase in density at other sites around their bodies.

How does soy perform this magic? First, isoflavones appear to increase your body's ability to hold onto the calcium you get from food and supplements. Second, isoflavones appear to preserve bone, as does estrogen, and build bone, as does testosterone.

Isoflavones and Calcium

The average adult human body, male or female, contains about 1,200 grams (nearly 3 pounds) of calcium, most of it packed away in bones and teeth. Calcium is also found in the fluid around your cells where it acts as an electrolyte, a particle that regulates the flow of liquid in and out of cells and facilitates the transmission of electrical impulses between nerve cells and muscle cells so that muscles move smoothly and do not go into spasm.

Every day, approximately 7,000 mg of calcium flow in and out of your bones to perform work throughout your body. To keep bones strong, you must take in enough dietary calcium to even out this ebb and flow, and it's vital that your body holds on to the calcium you take in.

Digesting and metabolizing protein requires calcium, some of which is then excreted as a waste product in your urine. As a general rule, the more protein you eat, the more calcium you lose. Nutritionists estimate that you give up about 1 mg of calcium for every 1 gram of protein you ingest, a reasonable explanation for the lower loss of bone among vegetarians than among people whose diet is high in animal protein foods such as meat, fish, and poultry. Additionally, substituting soy protein for protein from animal foods improves calcium retention because metabolizing soy protein requires less calcium than metabolizing protein from animal foods. A person whose primary source of protein is animal foods may lose up to 150 mg of calcium a day, while a person whose primary source of protein is soy products loses only 100 mg, a 33% difference.

In one pioneering study reported in the *Journal of Clinical Endocrinology* in 1988, volunteers were fed diets that provided exactly the same amount of nutrients except for the source of the protein: animal foods in one diet, soy in the other. Measuring protein loss, the researchers found that the people getting protein from animal products lost 50% more calcium per day than those whose protein came exclusively from soy.

Isoflavones and Bone Cells

Because soy isoflavones normally act like estrogen, you're right to assume that they stop the excess resorption of bone tissue. Osteoclasts, the cells that destroy bone, are powered by an enzyme called tyrosine kinase. Any chemical that inactivates tyrosine kinase will protect your bones. Unfortunately, most tryrosine kinase inhibitors are toxic. But here's one that's safe: genistein. Both in vitro (in laboratory vessels) and in vivo (in live animals), genistein stops osteoclasts right in their tracks. Add it to glass laboratory vessels containing osteoclasts, and the osteoclasts give up the ghost. Feed it to rats whose ovaries have been removed (which means they're producing much less bone-protective estrogen) and their bones get heavier, thanks to genistein's inhibition of bone resorption and stimulation of new bone growth.

Table 5-2 sums up the ways in which soy isoflavones protect your bones.

Table 5-2 Eating Soy Protects Bones Four Ways

1. Soy foods provide calcium.
2. Soy proteins reduce the amount of calcium lost through urination.
3. Soy enzyme inhibitors slow the resorption of bone tissue.
4. Soy isoflavones stimulate the production of new bone.

Now for a Brief Word About a Mysterious Bone Builder

One little known but interesting fact about soybeans is that their oil contains omega-3 fatty acids, a form of polyunsaturated fatty acids found primarily in fatty fish such as salmon. Omega-3 fatty acids, already credited with reducing your risk of heart attack, may also protect your bones. This information is so new that nobody is really sure exactly how it works. But you can bet there'll be more to come. In the meantime, it couldn't hurt to steam or stir-fry some salmon into your daily tofu, and double the value for your bones.

GETTING THE CALCIUM YOU NEED

Once upon a time, about ten years ago, nutrition scientists believed that once we achieved peak bone density in our middle 20s, we stopped absorbing calcium or building new bone. All that was left was to hold on tight to what we had and hope for the best. A couple of years later, the experts pushed the peak age up to the mid-30s, but they still saw the rest of life as a slippery slope, downhill all the way.

Today, the picture's changed. Several new nutritional strategies allow us not only to stop bone loss but maybe even increase our bone mass later in life. The first remedy is estrogen (see the previous sections). The second remedy is an estrogen alternative such as raloxifene (also discussed earlier). The third is calcium, including calcium from soy foods, plus two new partners, vitamin D and vitamin K.

How Much Calcium Do You Need?

As early as 1984, a National Institute of Health Conference Advisory Panel recommended raising the RDA for calcium for adult men and healthy women of child-bearing age to 1,000 mg, the RDA for postmenopausal women taking estrogen to 1,000 mg, and the RDA for postmenopausal women not using hormones to 1,500 mg.

These recommendations were confirmed in a 1994 NIH Consensus Statement on optimal calcium intake, and finally, in 1998, the National Academy of Sciences has set new, higher RDAs: 1,300 mg for boys and girls ages 9 to 18; 1,000 mg for men and women ages

19 to 50; and 1,200 mg for people over 51. One surprising discovery is the possibility that pregnant women and nursing mothers may not need more calcium than other women in their age group. Comparing body calcium levels for nursing mothers and those who were bottle-feeding, Heidi J. Kalkwarf, Ph. D., assistant professor of pediatrics at Children's Hospital Center, the University of Cincinnati, found that breast-feeding "changes a woman's calcium metabolism in ways that preserve and protect bone. No need for more."

The new calcium RDAs have evolved during the continuing revision of nutrition recommendations that has produced a new nutrition buzz word, the Dietary Reference Intake (DRI), an umbrella term embracing several categories of nutritional recommendations for vitamins, minerals, and other nutrients. The categories include:

Recommended Dietary Allowance (RDA), the amount that protects against deficiency;

Adequate Intake (AI), the recommended amount for nutrients for which no RDA has yet been set;

Estimated Average Requirement (EAR), the amount that meets the nutritional needs of half the people in any one group, such as teenage girls or people older than 70; and

Tolerable Upper Intake Level (UL), the highest amount considered unlikely to cause an adverse effect.

DRI is a "major leap forward in nutrition science," says Vernon Young of MIT, chair of the Institute of Medicine committee that established the concept. "Instead of emphasizing prevention of deficiency, we're now talking about the beneficial effects of healthy eating."

Table 5-3 shows the new categories of calcium recommendations.

Table 5-3 Calcium Recommendations

Age	RDA	AI	EAR*	UL
9–18	1,300	1,300	—	2,500
19–50	1,000	1,000	—	2,500
51+	1,200	1,200	—	2,500

*Not applicable

Source: National Academy Press, *Dietary Reference Intakes for Calcium Phosphorus, Magnesium, Vitamin D, and Fluoride* (Washington D.C., 1997).

BOOSTING CALCIUM UPTAKE WITH VITAMINS D AND K

Chemically, vitamin D is a steroid, a member of the same chemical family as estrogen. Like estrogen, vitamin D enables calcium to move into bones. That is why milk sold in the United States is fortified with vitamin D.

Because bone growth was previously assumed to be age-limited, vitamin D's benefits were also considered to be age-related. But in 1997, Bess Dawson-Hughes and several colleagues at the Jean Mayer U.S. Department of Agriculture Human Nutrition Research Center on Aging at Tufts University, came up with a new and intriguing possibility: Losing bone as we grow older may be due to inadequate supplies of vitamin D. For three years, Dawson asked 176 men and 2,134 women older than 65 to take either 500 mg of calcium plus 700 IU of vitamin D a day or a placebo.

At the end of one year, the men and women who took calcium and vitamin D had gained bone, while those on the placebo lost bone. At the end of three years, there was a significant difference in whole-body bone density between the two groups, and those on the placebo had suffered more than twice as many fractures as those on the mineral/vitamin pill. Based on these results, Dawson-Hughes says that future recommendations for vitamin D may rise to 600 mg/day for people older than 70, which is 200 mg above the current RDAs. But be warned: Doses of vitamin D exceeding 1,000 mg a day are considered hazardous.

A second calcium partner, vitamin K, activates at least three different proteins involved in the formation of bone tissue, says Johns Hopkins nutrition researcher Lori Sokoll, Ph. D. For example, one of these proteins, osteocalcin, needs to hook up with carbon-and-oxygen molecular fragments called "carboxyl groups" in order to build bone. This coupling is facilitated by vitamin K. When nine healthy volunteers at the Jean Mayer center in Boston took doses of vitamin K in an amount that was four times the RDA, their bodies produced more fully equipped osteocalcin, a development that researcher James A. Sadowski believes improves the outlook for their bone health. However, this is very preliminary information and further research is needed.

Calcium from Soy

Say "calcium," and most people think milk or dairy foods. And why not? As you can see from Table 5-4, milk and dairy foods are rich in calcium.

Table 5-4 Servings of Common Foods that Provide 250 mg of Calcium (or More)

Food	Serving	Calcium (mg)
Cheese		
Camembert	1 wedge	147
cottage, 2% fat	1 cup	155
Edam	1 oz	207
Gouda	1 oz	196
mozzarella, whole milk	1 oz	146
mozzarella, part skim	1 oz	183
Ice cream		
vanilla	½ cup	94
Milk		
whole milk	1 cup	291
2% milk	1 cup	297
skim milk	1 cup	302
Yogurt		
whole milk	1 cup	296
skim milk	1 cup	487

Source: USDA, *Composition of Foods*, USDA Handbook #8-16 (Washington D.C.).

But there's another group of foods that can serve up the calcium you need. From now on, whenever anyone says the C-word in your presence, think "soy." One cup of cooked soybeans provides about 18% of your RDA. Not a major amount, but again, every little bit helps. One cup of calcium-fortified soy milk gives you 25% to 30% of your RDA; and one 4-ounce serving of calcium-processed tofu, as much as 45%.

Table 5-5 lists the amount of calcium in representative servings of soy foods.

Food versus Supplements

Right about now, you're probably wondering whether it's okay to get the calcium you need from supplements rather than food. Surprise: The unequivocal answer is, yes.

No matter how often we are urged to include high-calcium foods in our diet, most Americans—especially young girls and women in their teens and early 20s—just don't get enough calcium from

Table 5-5 How Much Calcium Is in That Soy?

Food (amount)	Calcium (mg)
Soybeans, dried (½ cup)	80
Soybeans, green (½ cup)	130
Tempeh (4 ounces)	77
Tofu (4 ounces)	130*
Texturized soy protein (½ cup)	85
Soy milk (1 cup)	80
Soy milk, fortified (1 cup)	250–300

*Average; depending on processing, may contain 80–450 mg.

Source: United Soybean Board, *Soyfood for Thought*, #2, prepared by Mark Messina and Virginia Messina, n.d.

food. In fact, U.S. Department of Agriculture surveys show that few adult American women get more than 66% of the recommended dietary allowance of calcium from their food, and teenage girls do even worse.

I won't bother to go through the song and dance about how it's always better to get your nutrients from food rather than pills because food gives you vitamins and minerals, plus protein, fat, carbohydrates, and fiber. Nor will I belabor the point that you can get the calcium you need simply by juggling your diet to include a half cup of calcium-stiffened tofu here, a glass of calcium-fortified soy milk there, an ounce of cheese, a cup of yogurt, and so on until, practically before you know it, you've toted up 1,200 mg of calcium. The simple fact is that if you don't like these foods or you can't guarantee you'll get enough every day, calcium supplements are a fine substitute.

In fact, for many people, they are a necessity, says Bonnie Leibman, Director of Nutrition at the Center for Science in the Public Interest. Leibman recommends a daily multivitamin, multimineral supplement as low-cost health insurance, and *The Western Journal of Medicine* agrees. In a recent editorial the *Journal* editors said that an increased use of vitamin and mineral supplements could lower our national hospital bill by $20 billion, which would be due to a reduced rate of heart disease among people taking vitamin E and lower rates of birth defects and low-birth-weight infants among women taking multivitamins and minerals with folic acid and zinc. The other important supplement endorsed by Leibman is calcium. "You've got to take a separate pill," she says, "because a multi with a sufficient amount of calcium would be too bulky."

Ah, but which calcium to take? In nature, calcium is never found alone. It is always part of a chemical compound with another substance such as citric acid (calcium citrate), milk sugar (calcium lactate), chalk (calcium carbonate), and so on. As a result, calcium supplements come in a dizzying variety of compounds. The ones generally considered to be most easily absorbed by the body are calcium carbonate, calcium citrate, calcium citrate malate, and calcium phosphate.

Now, let's talk about how much calcium you're going to get from each pill. The amount of calcium in a calcium supplement is described in terms of "elemental calcium," the form in which it is absorbed by the body. For example, the label may say "500 mg of calcium carbonate providing 200 mg of elemental calcium."

Because calcium is best absorbed in doses of 500 mg or less, you get more calcium out of two 500-mg calcium tablets taken a couple of hours apart than you do from one 1,000-mg tablet. If there's a price break on the larger ones, buy them, then break them in half and take one half at a time. And increase your absorption of calcium from calcium carbonate by taking the tablets with meals.

Table 5-6 describes the various kinds of calcium in calcium supplements.

Table 5-6 The Calcium in Calcium Supplements

Calcium carbonate	=	a naturally occurring substance found in oyster shells and limestone
Calcium lactate	=	calcium plus lactic acid (the form of calcium in milk and dairy products)
Calcium citrate	=	calcium plus citric acid, the organic acid found in oranges, lemons, limes, and other fruit

Consumer alert: Calcium carbonate not only builds strong bones, it's also an antacid that soothes an upset stomach. The drug companies make hay with this by labeling calcium antacids as bone builders, too. But some antacids are made with magnesium or aluminum compounds rather than calcium carbonate. These products are fine for your stomach, but they won't help your bones. In fact, they may actually reduce your absorption of calcium, so check the label before you buy an antacid.

SUMMING UP

Soy phytoestrogens are as beneficial to your bones as they are to your heart. Just as they reduce your risk of some kinds of cancer, they also reduce your risk of osteoporosis by helping you to conserve bone density and build new bone tissue. Soy foods are a good source of calcium; 1 cup of soybeans or calcium-fortified soy milk has almost as much calcium as 1 cup of cow's milk. And best of all, this good medicine tastes great. Safe, effective—and tasty. Who could ask for anything more?

6

Hot News About Hot Flashes

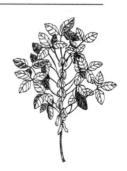

WHAT A HOT FLASH IS

Weaker bones aren't the only consequence of decreased estrogen secretion at menopause. The decline in estrogen also affects how your body regulates temperature, and that leads straight to one of the more unpleasant signs of menopause, the hot flash.

We are warm-blooded animals. We control our body temperature by dilating and constricting our blood vessels to regulate the flow of blood throughout our bodies. The temperature in the center of the body, where our organs are, is usually warmer than the temperature of our skin. When we feel chilled, our bodies will seek to protect their core warmth by constricting tiny blood vessels (capillaries) just under the skin so that less warm blood flows up to the skin and less chilled blood flows back into the center of the body. When we are very warm, the process reverses. The capillaries expand, and more warm blood flows up to the relatively cooler surface of the skin, then circulates back to cool our organs.

A hot flash (or hot flush) is a sudden feeling of intense heat over your face and upper body, which is sometimes accompanied by reddening of the skin and sweating. No one has yet conclusively identified the mechanism for hot flashes, but it is clearly related to an unpredictable dilation and constriction of the blood vessels. One theory pins the blame on a sudden release of a hormone called gonadotropin-releasing hormone (GRH) from your hypothalamus. The release of this hormone is your body's call for more estrogen. At menopause, when the estrogen is not forthcoming, areas of your brain that regulate your body temperature by controlling the dilation and constriction of blood vessels go haywire. The result is a hot flash.

Eight of every ten American women experience hot flashes at menopause, sometimes even before menstruation ends. Hot flashes tend to occur more often late in the day, after you eat or drink something hot, in hot weather, or at any time of the day (or year) when you are tense. For most of us, the frequency and intensity of the hot flashes tend to diminish within three to four years.

But here's a really interesting fact: The Japanese language doesn't even have a word for hot flashes. At the very least, this suggests either that hot flashes don't happen in Japan or that they are an extremely mild event. It's not much of a leap to think that one reason for this may be a diet rich in soy and soy phytoestrogens.

SOY AND HOT FLASHES

At the beginning of 1997, Gregory Burke, of the Department of Public Health at Bowman Gray School of Medicine in Winston-Salem, North Carolina, published the results of a small (43 women), 18-week study among volunteers ages 45 to 55 who were experiencing at least one hot flash a day. For the first six weeks, the women sprinkled 20 grams of soy protein over their cereal or mixed it into their juice at breakfast. For the second six weeks, they took 20 grams of soy divided into two doses each day. In the third six weeks they took a placebo, a powder that looked like soy protein but wasn't. While they were using the soy protein, the women all had significantly fewer hot flashes and night sweats. And as an added bonus, their cholesterol levels fell an average of 10%. Burke found these results so encouraging that he immediately set up a bigger study, this time with 240 women and larger servings of soy. While waiting for the results of this new effort, the Bowman Gray researchers cautiously advocate adding soy to your diet as an alternative to hormone-replacement therapy.

Meanwhile, across the Atlantic at University Hospital in South Manchester, England, breast cancer surgeon Nigel Bundred set up a study of his own, giving 30 Manchester women 60 grams of soy protein a day, three times the amount in the Bowman Gray study. The result was a significant reduction in the incidence (down 50%) and severity (300% less) of hot flashes.

Finally, halfway around the world, in Australia, a strong women's movement and its opposition to hormone therapy have supported a wealth of studies on natural alternatives to hormone therapy, including the use of soy rather than estrogen for hot flashes. In 1996, a team of Australians led by Alice Murkies of the Jean Hailes Centre for Women in Clayton, Victoria, decided to compare the anti–hot flash power of two different kinds of phytoestrogens, the isoflavones (daidzein and genistein) from soy versus the lignans in wheat. Murkies's study included 58 postmenopausal women, with an average age of 54, who were having at least 14 hot flashes a week. Half the women were given 28 grams of soy flour a day; the other half got 28 grams of wheat flour. In the end, both groups of women were experiencing fewer hot flashes, but the decline (40% fewer hot flashes) was greater for the women getting the soy than for those getting the wheat (25% fewer hot flashes). Unlike some earlier soy studies, this one produced no change in cholesterol levels.

Burke, Bundred, and Murkies gave their volunteers soy protein as powder or flour, not a terribly appetizing treat. But that doesn't mean you can't have your soy and enjoy it, too. Table 6-1 shows the grams of soy protein in representative servings of soy foods.

Another Soy Benefit

Yet another annoying sign of declining estrogen secretion at menopause is vaginal atrophy. Without sufficient estrogen, the tissues lining the vagina become thin and dry, and normal natural lubrication slows so that sexual intercourse may be painful, the lining of the vagina may actually tear, and vaginal infections are more common.

Hormone-replacement therapy cures vaginal atrophy. So does the local application of estrogen creams. But both, as you already know, also increase the risk of various kinds of reproductive cancers. So a second study from Alice Murkies and a group of Australians from the Monash Medical Centre, and the Royal Women's Hospital comparing the effects of phytoestrogens from soy, wheat, and linseed on 52 postmenopausal volunteers promises good news for older women.

Table 6-1 The Protein Content of Soy Foods

There is this much soy protein . . .	*. . . in this much soyfood*
20 grams	¾ cup cooked soybeans 3 cups soy milk ¼ cup roasted soybeans ⅔ cup soy flour ⅔ cup tempeh 1 cup tofu 1 cup (reconstituted) texturized soy protein
60 grams	2¼ cups cooked soybeans 9 cups soy milk ¾ cup roasted soybeans 2 cups soy flour 2 cups tempeh 3 cups tofu 3 cups (reconstituted) texturized soy protein

Source: United Soybean Board, Adapted from Soy Facts #5, *Soyfoods & Heart Disease* (n.d.).

The Aussies set up two 12-week trials. In the first, the volunteers were given daily servings of either 45 mg of soy grits with high concentrations of phytoestrogens or 45 grams of low-phytoestrogen wheat kibble. In the second trial, they got either 45 grams of linseed with a high concentration of phytoestrogens each day or 45 grams of the low-phytoestrogen wheat. As the study proceeded, the researchers counted hot flashes, examined vaginal cytology, and measured bone density and mineral content. In the end, the women who got the high-phytoestrogen foods not only excreted larger amounts of phytoestrogens in their urine (an expected result), they also showed a significant improvement in vaginal cytology. Before the study began, the maturation index of their vaginal cells (an indication of the number and health of functioning tissue cells) averaged 16. After the study ended, it was 33.

Women consuming soy grits also had a significant increase in bone mineral, a measurement of bone strength. Prior to the trial, they

Table 6-2 Comparing the Effects of Phytoestrogens on the Incidence of Hot Flashes

	Number of Daily Hot Flashes		
	Soy Grits	*Wheat Kibble*	*Linseed*
Before trial	5.06	5.75	5.75
During trial	3.93	2.97	3.39

Source: F. S. I. Dulais, et al. "Dietary Soy Supplementation Increases Vaginal Cytology Maturation Index and Bone Mineral Content in Postmenopausal Women." Second International Symposium on the Role of Soy in Preventing and Treating Chronic Disease (Brussels, September 15–18, 1996).

had averaged about 2,573 grams of bone mineral. Afterward, the average rose nearly 10%, to 2,713 grams. But the women who got wheat kibble and linseed did better in the hot flash department, scoring a greater decrease in the daily incidence of hot flashes. In the end, the researchers threw up their (figurative) hands, noting simply that this is the first study in humans to show a measurable increase in bone mineral content with increased soy intake.

Table 6-2 shows the results of the Murkies study demonstrating the effects of different kinds of phytoestrogens on the incidence of hot flashes.

OTHER PLANTS THAT MAY RELIEVE HOT FLASHES

Herbal medicine has a long and honored tradition of using plants to ameliorate signs of menopause such as hot flashes, but you should know that until recently there have been very few (translation: practically no) serious, controlled clinical trials of estrogenic plants in the United States.

In addition, until now there have been virtually no standards for labeling dietary supplements, the term used to describe a group of products that include those made from herbs. In 1998, the Food and Drug Administration announced new rules that require companies that make and market dietary supplements, including herbal products, to avoid making health claims. But, there is still no requirement for standardized dosages or a stipulation that manufacturers provide evidence of a product's safety and effectiveness. As a result, if you buy an aspirin or an antibiotic or a vitamin pill, you can be sure of the dose and be sure that the drug does what it's supposed to. After all, it's right there on the label. But herbal supplements cannot be marketed by making health claims, so there's no guarantee as to their potency or performance.

While we all wait anxiously for serious evaluations of herbal supplements, here is what we already know about three herbs often "prescribed" for hot flashes: black cohosh, dong quai, and red clover.

Black cohosh *(Cimicifuga racemosa)*, a.k.a. squaw root, black snake root, and tattle weed, is an herb that grows naturally in North American forests. American Indians boiled the root into a tea for a variety of "female problems" (hence, the name squaw root), and Lydia Pinkham used it in her famous Vegetable Compound. But the herb, once listed as an official drug in the U.S. Pharmacopoeia, is no longer used in medicine. Black cohosh's estrogenic effects may be due to a form of natural steroid compound called actein, which lowers blood pressure in some laboratory animals (rabbits, cats) and may—emphasize may—reduce levels of luteinizing hormone (LH), which are usually higher in menopausal women than they are in women who have not reached menopause.

Dong quai (Chinese angelica) is a perennial herb that is native to China and Japan, where it has long been used for menopausal or menstrual discomfort. Until recently, all of the studies on dong quai came from China. Fairly or not, they were not considered to have met the standards of Western medical research. Now, the first well-controlled Western study of dong quai, at Kaiser Permanente Medical Care Program of Northern California, has produced less-than-rave reviews. Seventy-one postmenopausal women with hot flashes or night sweats were randomly assigned to take either dong quai capsules or placebos three times a day for 24 weeks. In the end, there were no significant differences between the two groups, either in terms of the severity of their hot flashes or the levels of estrogen in their blood, so the Kaiser Permanente researchers rated the dong quai to be no more effective than a placebo. Nevertheless, they were careful to point out that this study does not necessarily mean that dong quai cannot be effective in treating hot flashes. In the United State, they note, dong quai is usually sold alone, as a single ingredient product. In China, it is used in combination with other herbs, and that may be the key to its effectiveness.*

However, a study by Catherine L. Eagon, a physician at Allegheny General Hospital in Pittsburgh, and her sister, Patricia K. Eagon, a biochemist at the University of Pittsburgh, suggests an alternative possibility. The Eagons, systematically examining the effectiveness of herbal remedies for hot flashes, stirred extracts of dong quai into test tubes containing cells with estrogen receptor sites. They found that molecules of dong quai, as well as molecules of licorice root (*Glycyrrhiza uralensis*) and blue cohosh (*Caulophyllum thalictroides*)—but not black cohosh—were actively attracted to the sites.

The third herb that is thought to reduce the severity of hot flashes is red clover, a plant that contains formononetin, a phytoestrogen that is also found in soybeans. In your body, formononetin is converted to daidzein, and that may be the secret of red clover's reputation as a menopause tonic.

Early in 1998, John Eden, of the Department of Obstetrics and Gynecology at the University of New South Wales, Australia, set up a 12-week study in which he randomly assigned 40 menopausal volunteers to one of three treatment regimens—40 mg of red clover extract (as Promensil, an over-the-counter product), 160 mg of red clover extract (Promensil), or a placebo. At the end of the trial, says Eden, "the women who were able to absorb sufficient daidzein as measured by the amount of daidzein excreted in their urine had a significant improvement in their hot flushes."

---

*At Columbia University's Rosenthal Center for Complementary and Alternative Medicine in New York, researcher Fredi Kronenberg is currently running a double-blind study with 40 women who are taking a mixture of 10 Chinese herbs (other than dong quai) in an effort to evaluate their effectiveness in relieving hot flashes. Kronenberg's data was expected to be ready by the summer of 1998, too late to include in this book but not too late for you to check your newspaper for the results.

Note: A single-blind study is one in which the researchers know who is getting the substance being evaluated and who is getting the placebo. In a double-blind study, neither the volunteers nor the researchers know who is getting what. Therefore, a double-blind study is regarded as being the most bias-free kind of research.

Data from Eden's study should be published just as this book reaches your bookstore. Promensil is already on sale here in the United States. Anecdotal evidence in the form of reports by women who have used red clover extract suggest that it provides some relief from hot flashes, but there are still no studies to attest to its safety in long-term use. In fact, this is a problem with virtually every herbal remedy for hot flashes, and, as Patricia Eagon notes, women using these herbals should think of them not as harmless foods, but as powerful medicines.

VITAMINS, MINERALS, AND HOT FLASHES

It is increasingly obvious that the nutritional needs of older women, and older men, too, differ from those of younger people. The last RDAs, written nearly ten years ago, lumped everyone older than 51 into one category, but that's about to change. The RDAs that are in the works for 1999 are likely to separate the "near-old" from the "old" and the "very old."

It's about time. As more of us live to a ripe old age, there's been a virtual explosion of research into the effects of diet on longevity and good health. For example, we've learned that vitamin and mineral supplements can protect aging eyes, minds, and immune systems, while lowering the age-related risk of cancer and heart disease.

- Data from the Harvard/Brigham Women's Hospital Nurses Health Study hints that long-term use of vitamin C supplements (400–700 mg/day) can slow chemical reactions that cause proteins in the lens of the eye to clump together, forming cataracts that cloud the lens and dim our vision. In a separate study, the antioxidant carotenoid lutein (a yellow pigment in spinach and green leafy vegetables) appears to protect the retina of your eye from macular degeneration, an age-related condition that can cause partial blindness. "Follow-up studies should shed more light on how these nutrients work," puns Julie Mares-Perlman, Ph. D., assistant professor of ophthalmology at the University of Wisconsin Medical School.
- In Madrid, a 1997 University of Complutens' review of the diets of 260 healthy Madrid men and women ages 60 to 90 finds that

those who eat foods rich in vitamin E, vitamin C, folic acid, dietary fiber, and complex carbohydrates scored high on cognitive tests. "In an aging population, a diet high in antioxidants and low in fat preserves thinking processes and memory," says study leader Rosa M. Ortega.

- Moderate doses of vitamin E also boost the elderly person's immune system. In Boston, when USDA researcher Simin Nikbin Meydani, Ph.D., D.V.M., gave 80 healthy senior citizens a daily pill containing either 60, 200, or 800 mg of vitamin E or a placebo, those taking 200 mg had the best response: a 65% increase in the activity of T cells, immune system cells that "remember" an invader (such as a virus) and how to beat it. "Our next study," she says, "will test whether this means better protection against colds."

- Nutritionists once believed that our bodies did not absorb calcium or build bone density after our middle 20s. Today—even though it is still considered vital to accumulate bone mass while we are young—it's clear that increasing and maintaining calcium consumption as we grow older reduces the age-related loss of bone that leads to osteoporosis. This is particularly important for women who do not wish to take hormone-replacement therapy.

- As for heart disease, the major killer of older women, studies show that the B vitamin folate (folic acid, folacin) may reduce the risk of heart attack by lowering blood levels of the amino acid homocysteine; this suggests that increasing the amount of folates we get from our diets or adding a B vitamin supplement may offer added protection.

Unfortunately, most of what we think we know about the value of vitamins and minerals in relieving hot flashes is still anecdotal ("My best friend's sister tried this when she hit menopause and she says that . . .") rather than scientific.

More than 50 years ago, a 1945 article in the *American Journal of Obstetrics and Gynecology* said that vitamin E supplements could help relieve hot flashes and vaginal atrophy. Four years later, there was a study of 66 women, half of whom said their hot flashes and dry skin improved when they took 20 to 100 IU of vitamin E a day. Since then, we've learned that vitamin E can protect the heart, but its effects on the skin and on hot flashes are still unproven.

To date, there simply have not been any rigorously controlled trials comparing the reactions of women taking vitamin E to a control group given a look-alike pill. However, unless you have high blood pressure or another problem that your doctor says mitigates against your taking this vitamin, E is considered a safe supplement. The usual "dose" for hot flashes is 800–1,200 IU, much higher than the current RDA (40 IU).

Because vitamin B_6 (pyridoxine) plays a role in the body's production of sex hormones, including estrogen, some women believe that it is valuable for hot flashes. There is no proof that this is true, and, unlike vitamin E, vitamin B_6 is not free of potentially serious side effects. It is considered nontoxic in amounts up to 20 mg (10 times the 2.0 mg RDA for men; more than 10 times the 1.6 mg RDA for women), but larger doses, starting at 50 mg a day, have been reported to damage peripheral nerves, the nerves in arms and legs, hands and feet. This effect was first widely reported among women using gram doses of vitamin B_6 (amounts in excess of 1,000 mg) to relieve menstrual discomfort or pain from carpal tunnel syndrome.

The Bottom Line on Nutrients

While vitamins and minerals (with the exception of calcium) have yet to be proven effective in alleviating or reversing the signs of menopause, they can be invaluable in maintaining health and vibrancy as we grow older. Older Americans often do not eat as well as they should. They may live alone and may hate to cook for one person. Their fixed incomes may not stretch to cover a wide variety of healthful foods. They may not have the appetite they once enjoyed because they are not as active. Or they may simply forget to eat. All these things are reasons for choosing a good, basic, RDA-level vitamin and mineral supplement to keep your body in nutritional balance.

SIMPLE LIFESTYLE CHANGES

Not everything in life requires a medical solution. Sometimes simply altering small details in our lives can produce big results. For example, here are some way to reduce the discomfort of hot flashes without medicine, herbs, or even vitamins.

Change Your Clothes

It's simple physics. If you're having hot flashes, you'll be more comfortable in breathable fabrics that keep you cool and allow moisture (that's sweat) to evaporate from your skin. The ultimate hot-flash-friendly fabric is cotton, as in cotton knit T-shirts, cotton knit dresses, and cotton sweaters. Linen is good, too. So is silk, although it stains easily.

Layering is a wonderfully protective technique. When the hot flash hits, you can peel off the jacket or vest, then put it back on when things cool off. Give your favorite, but uncomfortable, wool clothes to a younger relative or the local neighborhood women's shelter. Don't you feel cooler just thinking about that?

Change Your Mind

Meditation, bio-feedback, and other relaxation techniques can actually make you feel cooler all over by teaching you how to influence processes such as the dilation and constriction of your blood vessels, an autonomic bodily function that was once considered beyond conscious control. Sometimes just concentrating on feeling cooler does the trick. Don't ask me how it works. All I know is that having tried it myself, starting as a total skeptic, my best advice echoes that old commercial: Try it. You may like it.

Change Your Diet

Some women find that their hot flashes worsen when they drink coffee, tea, or sodas containing caffeine; use alcoholic beverages; eat high-fat foods or foods with "hot" spices, such as curry or peppers; or serve up very hot (temperature-wise) dishes and beverages.

They have a point. Or several. Caffeine, alcohol, and the phyto-chemicals in hot spices all affect blood vessels' dilation and contraction. If this fits your experience, why not perform a simple experiment? Try a week or two without any of these foods. If eliminating them from your diet reduces the number and severity of your hot flashes, you have your answer. Then, to identify the offending food(s), just add them back, one at a time, to see which one sets off the hot flashes.

SUMMING UP

Because soy and soy foods contain phytoestrogens, it is logical to think that they might relieve signs of menopause, such as hot flashes and vaginal atrophy, due to your body's declining secretion of natural estrogens. A growing body of research suggests that this may indeed be true, but right now there is no conclusive proof. The same may be said for herbal remedies, as well as vitamins and minerals. Because these remedies are considered safe there's no reason not to try them. Think of yourself as the Marie Curie of your own personal menopause.

7

Cooking with Soy

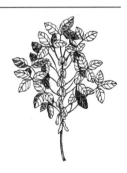

The Joy of Soy

I challenge you to think of a food that is more versatile than the simple soybean. Not only does it yield up a multiplicity of different products—basic beans, soy flour, soy milk, soybean oil, and three meat substitutes (tofu, tempeh, and texturized soy protein)—it's also the King of the Culinary Chameleons, adaptable to virtually any dish and, given some care, pleasing to practically every palate.

This chapter is a short, introductory guide to cooking with soy. Because preparing food is an intensely personal art, many of the recipes you'll find here are either ones I am accustomed to using in my own kitchen, or my adaptations of recipes that intrigued me, or dishes I've sampled in other homes or in restaurants.

I am indebted to the Soyfoods Association of America's United Soybean Board (USB) for their kind permission to reprint several of their delicious recipes, developed by the Soyfoods Association of America. Each of these recipes is identified with an asterisk (*). For more recipes and tips on how to use soy products, you may call the USB information line, 1-800-TALK-SOY, or check out its website at www.talksoy.com.

Recipes marked with a plus sign (+) come from the Indiana Soybean Board, which has graciously granted me permission to reprint them. A third source of soy food recipes and info is the USB/University of Illinois soy information website (www.ag.uiuc.edu/~stratsoy/soyhealth/).

At the end of most recipes, you will find the amount of soy protein and soy isoflavones per serving. These amounts, which are only approximate, are based on Table 1-8 (Protein Content of Common Foods) and Table 2-3 (The Isoflavone Content of Soy Foods).

Now let's start to build your soy repertory with whole beans, either edamame, the fresh, green beans you can use as a vegetable or side dish; dried beans, for a hearty main entry; or roasted into "soy nuts." Use tempeh, that deep, rich, flavorful cake of roasted soybeans, instead of meat on the grill or in your stews. Make burgers, meatballs, or meatloaf from texturized soy protein. Season your soups with miso. Use soy sauce instead of salt on fish, chicken, and beef. Serve soy grits instead of rice. Bake with soy flour. Spread soy nut butter on your soy bread. Savor the flavor and "mouth-feel" of cholesterol-free dairy substitutes such as soy milk, soy cheese, soy yogurt, or a rich, creamy frozen soy dessert. Sauté tofu with veggies or whip it into salad dressings and dips—and, yes, even a chocolate cream pie. Then wash it all down with a soy beverage. *Salut!*

WHOLE SOYBEANS

Whole soybeans are available fresh, dried, or canned. The cream-colored canned beans are ready to use right from the package; fresh beans are prepared like any other vegetables; dried beans must be soaked before cooking.

Fresh soybeans, also known as edamame, are generally sold in Asian food markets where you may find them fresh or frozen, in the pod like ordinary green peas, or shelled. The beans must always be refrigerated and should be used within a day or two after purchase. Frozen green soybeans stay fresh in the freezer for several months.

Dried mature soybeans, creamy tan to light yellow in color, come packed in plastic bags or loose in bins. Given the choice, I would opt for the bagged beans because the plastic protects them from air, dirt, and insects.

Like other dried beans, dried soybeans must be "precooked" before using. The first step is to figure out the quantity of beans you will need for your recipe. (As a general rule, 1 cup of dried, uncooked soybeans equals 2 to 3 cups of cooked beans.) Next, put the dried soybeans into a colander and "pick them over." Take out small pebbles and any other debris. Once that's done, rinse the beans under cool, running water, and put them in a large pot. Add water, about 6 cups of water to 1 pound of beans. Now either cover the pot and let it sit overnight, or bring the water to a fast boil for 1 minute, turn off the flame, and let the beans sit for 1 hour. After the beans have soaked overnight or for an hour, drain, rinse, and use them as directed in your recipe. (Note: The quantities of dried soybeans listed in the following recipes are measured after pre-cooking.)

Finally, here's a nifty bonus to cooking soybeans. As you simmer the fresh or dried beans in water, the air in your kitchen will slowly fill with the wonderful aroma of—get this!—chicken soup. It's another lovely surprise from a wonderful food.

Roasted Soybeans

1 tablespoon soy oil
1 teaspoon salt
4 cloves garlic, minced

1 teaspoon chili powder
3 cups precooked dried soybeans

Preheat the oven to 350 degrees. Lightly oil a large cookie sheet. Combine the salt, garlic, and chili powder. Spread the precooked beans over the cookie sheet, then sprinkle them with the seasoning mixture. Bake the beans for 1 hour or until lightly browned, shaking the pan lightly every 15 minutes to keep them from sticking. Serve warm or cool.

Yield: 3 cups of soy nuts

Soy protein: 28 g per cup
Soy isoflavones: 70 mg per cup

Savory Baked Beans (*)

2   pounds whole dried
    soybeans
6   cups water
¾   cup dark molasses
½   cup packed brown sugar
1   tablespoon dry mustard
1   tablespoon tamari or
    soy sauce

¼   teaspoon cayenne pepper
1   teaspoon pepper (black or
    white, ground)
1   large onion, chopped
½   cup green pepper, chopped
3   cloves garlic, minced
2   bay leaves
½   teaspoon cloves (whole)

Soak and precook the whole dried soybeans.

Preheat the oven to 300 degrees. Combine all of the ingredients in a large, covered, ovenproof bean pot or casserole and bake for 7 to 8 hours. Check them periodically and add more water, as needed, to prevent the beans from burning. The beans are done when tender. Serve with brown bread as a main dish or with your favorite meal as a side dish.

Yield: up to 16 servings, depending on size

Soybean Cioppino (Fish Stew)

1   tablespoon olive oil
¼   cup (each) diced carrots
       and onions
2   cloves garlic, diced
1   (14-ounce) can whole
       tomatoes (about seven),
       drained and chopped plus
       1 cup tomato liquid
4   cups water
1   large white potato, peeled
       and diced
⅔   cup precooked dried
       soybeans
1   cup finely sliced cabbage

½   cup diced summer squash
       (green or yellow)
2   teaspoons fennel seed
¼   teaspoon dried thyme
½   teaspoon dried basil
1   pound fresh cod, or 1 pound
       large shrimp, or 20 small
       clams, or any combination
       of fish
4   thick slices Italian or
       French bread
    Salt and pepper to taste
    Grated Parmesan cheese

Combine the olive oil, carrots, onions, and garlic in a large, heavy stewpot. Cover and cook over medium heat until the vegetables are soft, but not brown, about 10–15 minutes. Add the tomatoes, tomato liquid, water, potato, soybeans, cabbage, squash, fennel, thyme, and basil. Simmer for 1 hour. Check periodically and add water as needed.

Rinse the fish under cold water and cut into large chunks. Add it to the stew, bring it to a slow boil, and cook for 15 minutes. If using shellfish, add and simmer the stew 3 to 5 minutes, until shellfish become opaque.

Put one slice of bread into each of four soup plates. Use a slotted spoon to lift the fish and vegetables into a dish. Add salt and pepper to the liquid, then ladle the liquid over the stew. Top with grated Parmesan cheese.

Yield: 4 servings

Soy protein: 5 g per serving
Soy isoflavones: 12 mg per serving

Soybean, Carrot, and Potato Stew

8	whole medium carrots	1	teaspoon chili powder
1	tablespoon canola oil	1	tablespoon ancho pepper
2	large white onions, sliced		puree (see below)
2	cups precooked dried	1	teaspoon salt (or to taste)
	soybeans	1	large white potato, peeled
5	cups water		and sliced thick

Put the carrots in a small roasting dish, add oil, and roast for 25 minutes. Add the onion slices and roast for another 15 minutes. Remove from oven, slice the carrots into rounds, and put the carrots, onions, and beans in a stewpot with 5 cups water. Add chili powder, ancho pepper puree, and salt. Simmer for 1 hour, checking from time to time, and add water as needed to prevent the vegetables from sticking or burning. Add the potato and simmer for 1 hour, again adding water as needed. When the carrots and potatoes are tender, serve the dish as soup, a side dish, or a main dish with rice.

To make ancho pepper puree: Split one ancho pepper and remove the seeds. Flatten the pepper in a frying pan and heat it until it smokes, then turn and cook it on the other side. Put the cooked pepper in a bowl, cover it with boiling water, and soak it for ½ hour. Pour off the soaking water, and puree the pepper with ¼ cup of fresh warm water in a food processor, then rub the puree through a fine strainer and discard the solids. This may be prepared a day or two in advance and refrigerated.

Yield: 4 main dish servings; 8 or more side dish servings

Soy protein: 14 g per serving
Isoflavones: 38 mg per serving

Soybean Gumbo (*)

2   tablespoons soybean oil
½   cup chopped onions
2   cloves garlic, minced
2   tablespoons soy flour
2   tablespoons all-purpose
     flour
2   quarts vegetable, fish, or
     chicken stock
2   cups precooked soybeans
1   can (14½ ounces) cut okra,
     drained
2   cans (14½ ounces each)
     whole tomatoes

1   cup diced green pepper
1   teaspoon dried thyme,
     crushed
1   teaspoon salt
¼   to ½ teaspoon cayenne
     pepper
¼   teaspoon ground pepper
½   pound medium shrimp,
     cooked and peeled
4   to 6 cups cooked white rice

Heat the oil in a large, heavy stewpot. Add the onions and garlic and sauté until the onions are tender. Mix the flours together with ½ cup of stock; gradually stir the flour mixture into the onions to form a smooth, thin paste. Add the soybeans, okra, tomatoes (with liquid), green pepper, thyme, salt, cayenne pepper, ground pepper, and the remaining stock. Bring it to a boil, then reduce the heat and simmer it for 10 minutes. Add the shrimp and simmer the mixture another 5 minutes or until the shrimp have turned pink/white and are thoroughly cooked. Serve over rice.

Yield: 4 servings as a main dish; 8 servings as a first course

Soy protein: 14 g per main dish serving; 7 g per first course serving
Isoflavones: 38 mg per main dish serving; 19 mg per first course serving

Edamame (Green Soybean) Side Dish

1 pound fresh green soybeans
      in the pod or ½ pound shelled beans
   Seasonings (suggested
      seasonings listed below)

Open the pods, push out the beans, and discard the pods. Bring water to a boil in a large saucepan, add the beans, bring the water back to a boil, then turn it down to simmer, and cook the beans 10 to 15 minutes (or until tender).

   Season with chopped onions, chives, thyme, rosemary, cumin, or curry and serve as a side dish. Or, add the cooked beans to soups or salads.

Yield: 4 small servings

Edamame Snacks

1 pound fresh green
      soybeans in the pod

Simmer the beans in their pods (with or without salt and seasonings) for 10 to 15 minutes. Cool them to room temperature, and serve them in a bowl or dish. To eat, open the pods, and push out the cooked beans.

Yield: Variable

Tofu

Say "soy," and most Americans probably think of tofu, the bland, white, cheese-like food made from the liquid squeezed out of soybeans and stiffened with a firming agent such as gluconolactone, calcium chloride, or calcium sulfate.

Tofu comes in several consistencies. Silken tofu is creamy and custard-like. Soft tofu is slightly stiffer; firm is stiffer still; and extra firm is the stiffest of all. Each is a relatively low-fat, cholesterol-free protein food. Tofu thickened with a calcium compound is also an exemplary non-dairy source of calcium.

The simplest way to use tofu is to slice a firm or extra-firm block into cubes and serve it with a dipping sauce made of soy sauce with a splash of spiced oil and some sliced green onions (scallions) or green onions plus minced garlic. Or you can sauté the firm or extra-firm cubes with sliced green onions, diced red bell peppers, and minced garlic, then season them with soy sauce, and serve them over rice. Or how about an entire block of extra-firm tofu brushed with teriyaki sauce, roasted until browned, and then sliced to serve with rice and veggies?

In more complicated cookery, tofu's greatest virtue may be its ability to soak up the dominant flavor of any dish to which you add it. For example, instead of using 1 pound of beef cubes in a beef stew, use ¼ pound of beef cubes plus 12 ounces of extra-firm tofu cut into cubes. The flavor will still be rich and surprisingly meaty, but the fat and cholesterol content of the dish will be as much as 75% less. Ditto for scrambled eggs made with silken tofu; just substitute 12 ounces of tofu for four of the six eggs to make breakfast for three. Silken tofu is also a super stand-in for sour cream or yogurt in dips and a velvety base for a rich "cream" pie, as you will see in a following recipe.

Tofu comes packaged or in water-filled bins. As with whole beans, I'd choose the packaged version. At home, store tofu in the refrigerator, and once you open the package, use it within a few days. You can also freeze tofu for up to five months. Freezing tofu changes its color and may actually make it more tasty in mixed dishes. Defrosted frozen tofu is caramel-colored rather than pale creamy white, and it's more spongy, which means it soaks up more sauce and flavorings.

Tofu Chip Dip

1 (12-ounce) package firm tofu
     (for a firm dip) or silken tofu
     (for a smoother dip)
1 packet any flavor dip ingredients
     or dry salad dressing mix

Process or blend the tofu with the other ingredients. Chill it for several hours and serve.

Yield: Approximately 1 cup dip

Soy protein: 36 g per cup (firm tofu); 14.4 g per cup (silken tofu)
Soy isoflavones: 120 mg per cup

Tofu Sandwich Spread

4 ounces firm tofu	¼ cup chopped green onions
4 ounces large-curd cottage cheese	¼ cup chopped red pepper

Mash the tofu with the cottage cheese. Stir in the vegetables. Spread the mixture on bagels, rolls, or bread (preferably whole wheat, for a more intense flavor combination).

Yield: 2 sandwiches, depending on size

Soy protein: 7 g per sandwich
Soy isoflavones: 20 mg per sandwich

Pasta with Tofu and Chicken

1   tablespoon olive oil
4   chicken roaster legs, without the skin
2   large onions, sliced
3   cloves garlic, sliced
2   cups crushed tomatoes
1   cup water
2   large carrots, sliced thin
4   large white mushrooms, sliced thick
½   teaspoon sugar
1   tablespoon dried oregano
1   tablespoon dried basil
1   tablespoon fennel seed
1   pound extra-firm tofu, cut in cubes
    Salt, to taste
1   pound spaghetti or other pasta
    Grated Parmesan cheese

Pour the oil into a large, heavy saucepan and heat it gently. Add the skinless chicken legs and brown them on all sides, turning frequently to prevent sticking. Add the onions and garlic, cooking until the onions are translucent but not browned. Add all of the remaining ingredients except the tofu, salt, spaghetti, and cheese, and simmer gently for an hour, or until the chicken is tender and browned. Check often, adding water as needed to keep the sauce thick and to prevent sticking.

When the chicken is done and the sauce is thick, add the tofu chunks and salt to taste, then simmer the mixture for another 15 minutes. While the sauce is simmering, cook the pasta. Serve the sauce over the pasta, topped with Parmesan cheese.

Yield: 4 servings

Soy proteins: 13 g per serving
Soy isoflavones: 40 mg per serving

Grilled Tofu

1 pound firm tofu
1 teaspoon soy oil (plain or spiced)
2 tablespoons tamari soy sauce

Brush the tofu block with oil and coat it with tamari sauce on both sides. Place the block on a well-oiled grill or in the broiler or on a lightly oiled skillet and cook until golden brown on both sides.

Slice and serve it over rice, with chopped green onions and red bell peppers; or slice and combine it with grilled vegetables, as a sandwich filling for a pita bread; or use it on a tossed green salad.

Yield: 2 servings as main dish; 4 sandwiches or salads

Soy protein: 26 g per serving as main dish; 13 g per sandwich or salad
Soy isoflavones: 80 mg per serving as main dish; 20 mg per sandwich or salad

Tofu Meatloaf or Burgers

6 ounces firm tofu
1 pound lean chopped beef
1 tablespoon grated onion
1 teaspoon mixed herbs (basil, parsley, oregano, thyme)
1 teaspoon salt
¼ cup tomato catsup or tomato sauce

Preheat the oven to 350 degrees. Crumble the tofu and mix it thoroughly with the chopped beef, grated onion, herbs, and salt. Form the mixture into a meatloaf or 8 burgers. Brush catsup or tomato sauce over the top. Bake the meatloaf for 1 hour, or broil the burgers until done.

Yield: 8 servings

Soy protein: 2.5 g per serving
Soy isoflavones: 7.5 mg per serving

Dark Chocolate Tofu Pie

Crust

3 whole plain graham crackers
1 teaspoon unsalted margarine
  or
1 (8-inch) prepared graham
  cracker pie crust

Filling

2 pounds silken tofu
½ cup sugar
¼ cup skim milk
2 tablespoons unsalted
  margarine
½ cup plain, unsweetened
  cocoa powder
¼ teaspoon instant coffee or
  espresso powder
1 teaspoon vanilla

Preheat the oven to 350 degrees. Crush the graham crackers, melt the margarine, and combine. Press the crumbs onto the bottom of an 8-inch spring form pan, and bake for 10 minutes. Remove from the oven and set aside to cool. Turn the oven down to 325 degrees.

While the crust is cooling, drain the tofu and blend it with the other filling ingredients until smooth, using either an electric mixer or a food processor. Pour the filling into the pie shell. Bake for 50 minutes or until a toothpick/tester inserted in the center comes out clean. Remove the pie from the oven, chill for several hours, top with whipped cream (optional), and serve.

Yield: 8 small or 4 medium servings

Soy protein: 9.6 per small serving; 19 per large serving
Soy isoflavones: 40 mg per small serving; 80 mg per large serving

Tofu/Banana Drink

4   ounces silken tofu
1   medium banana, sliced
1   teaspoon sugar or artificial
      sweetener

$\frac{1}{4}$ teaspoon vanilla
5   ice cubes

Put all of the ingredients in a blender and process until smooth.

Yield: 1 serving

Soy protein: 9.6 g per serving
Soy isoflavones: 40 mg per serving

TEMPEH

Tempeh is a dense, chewy food made by adding a starter (fermenting agent) to a mixture of whole soybeans and grain, usually rice. Plain tempeh has a rich flavor that is sometimes described as smoky or nut-like or rather like mushrooms. Tempeh is also available with flavoring, such as "barbecue."

Like soybeans, tempeh benefits from pre-cooking, which in this case means a short session in the steamer. Cut the tempeh in cubes, pop it in your steamer for 5 to 7 minutes, then add the cubes to stews, spaghetti sauces, sloppy joes, soups, or casseroles. Like tofu, tempeh takes on the dominant flavor of the dish. Unlike tofu, which is utterly bland, even plain tempeh adds a few notes of its own for emphasis and it definitely deepens the natural mushroom flavor of any mushroom dish. Tempeh also adds a chewy meat-like texture to vegetarian cooking. It grills well and can be served up on skewers with vegetables. Just brush it with barbecue sauce and broil.

You can find tempeh in the frozen food section at your health food or Asian food store. At home, store it in the refrigerator and use within a week. Like other fermented products such as cheese, tempeh often has a bit of white mold on the surface. Not to worry: It's harmless.

Marinated Tempeh Kebabs (*)

Marinade
2   tablespoons lemon juice
2   tablespoons olive oil
¼   cup tamari
¼   cup tarragon vinegar
3   tablespoons mixed dried
      herbs (any combination of
      basil, oregano, thyme,
      rosemary, etc.)
3   cloves garlic, crushed
      Pepper to taste

Kebabs
8   ounces tempeh, cut into
      8 cubes
12   medium white mushrooms
1   sweet red pepper, cut into
      8 pieces
1   medium onion, quartered
1   small zucchini, cut into
      8 pieces

Combine marinade ingredients in a jar, shake well, and set aside. Put the tempeh cubes to steam over boiling water for 10 minutes.

Prepare the vegetables. Put the vegetables and steamed tempeh in large bowl, add the marinade, toss the mixture to coat the tempeh and veggies, and then refrigerate for at least 1 hour.

Arrange the tempeh and vegetables on 4 skewers and grill for 10 to 15 minutes, turning frequently and brushing with marinade. Serve with rice if desired.

Yield: 4 servings

Soy protein: 8.5 g per serving
Soy isoflavones: 20 mg per serving

Spicy Tempeh with Broccoli (*)

1 cup water	5 cups sliced broccoli
$\frac{1}{4}$ cup soy sauce	1 cup sliced mushrooms
1 tablespoon Szechuan sauce	1 cup sliced onion
1 tablespoon cornstarch	1 tablespoon soybean oil
1 teaspoon sugar	2 cups cooked rice
1 (8-ounce) package plain tempeh, cut in slices $1\frac{1}{2}$ x $\frac{1}{4}$ inches	

Combine the water, soy sauce, Szechuan sauce, cornstarch, and sugar. Mix well to dissolve the cornstarch and set aside.

Stir-fry the tempeh, broccoli, mushrooms, and onion with oil in a non-stick pan until the broccoli is crisp/tender. Add the liquid and cook 1 minute, stirring constantly until the sauce thickens. Serve over rice.

Yield: 4 servings

Soy protein: 8.5 g per serving
Soy isoflavones: 20 mg per serving

Tempeh/Chicken Curry

4	large chicken legs	½	cup raisins
1	tablespoon olive oil	1	(8-ounce) package of plain tempeh, cubed
2	large yellow onions, sliced		
3	cloves garlic, sliced	1	cup steamed cauliflower florets (optional)
1	to 2 teaspoons curry powder		
1	tablespoon dried oregano	2	white potatoes, peeled and cubed (optional)
1	teaspoon cumin		
1	cup chicken stock, or vegetable stock, or water	2	cups cooked Basmati rice
			Salt to taste
1	large Granny Smith apple, peeled and sliced		

Brown the chicken legs in a large saucepan with the oil, turning them frequently to avoid burning. Add the sliced onions and garlic and cook until the onions are translucent but not browned. Add the curry powder, oregano, and cumin; stir to mix them with the chicken and vegetables. Add stock or water, apples, and raisins and cook for 45 minutes, checking frequently and adding water as needed to prevent sticking.

Steam the tempeh cubes for 10 minutes, and add them to the curry with the steamed cauliflower florets and potatoes. Continue cooking for another 15 minutes or until the chicken is tender and browned. Serve with rice and salt to taste.

Yield: 4 servings.

Soy protein: 8.5 g per serving
Soy isoflavones: 20 mg per serving

Tempeh in Curry Cream Sauce

1 (8-ounce) package plain tempeh, cubed

1 tablespoon instant dry nonfat milk

1 cup vegetable stock or water

1 teaspoon butter or margarine or canola oil

1 large white onion, thinly sliced

1 tablespoon white flour

½ teaspoon cumin

1 teaspoon mild curry powder

¼ cup frozen peas

2 cups cooked Basmati rice

Steam the tempeh cubes for 10 minutes and set them aside. Dissolve the milk powder in the vegetable stock or water and set it aside. Warm the butter in a 2-quart saucepot. Add the onions and cook until they are translucent but not browned. Add the flour, cumin, and curry to the onions, stir quickly to coat, and immediately add the milk mixture, pouring slowly and stirring constantly to make a smooth sauce. Add the tempeh and peas, stirring to thicken the sauce, and heat the entire mixture. Serve over rice, with chutney.

Yield: 2 main dishes or 4 side dishes

Soy protein: 17 g per main dish serving; 8.5 g per side dish serving
Soy isoflavones: 40 mg per main dish serving; 20 mg per side dish serving

TEXTURIZED SOY PROTEIN (TSP)

Texturized soy protein is made of fat-free soy flour cooked and then extruded (pushed through a device that shapes it into granules or flakes). TSP granules and flakes are most commonly used in commercial food products, but they are also available for home use as a substitute for ground beef. TSP also comes formed into chunks that can be added to stews and soups.

The first step in using TSP is to put back the moisture that was removed when the flour was defatted and cooked. You do this by adding ⅞ cup of hot water to 1 cup of TSP granules or flakes, stirring, and then letting the mixture sit for a few minutes until the liquid is absorbed. To rehydrate TSP chunks, simmer them in hot water for several minutes, as directed on the package.

For "formed" chopped meat dishes such as meatloaf, meatballs, and burgers, replace ¼ of the beef with TSP. In highly seasoned, "loose meat" dishes such as sloppy joes, beef stroganoffs, chili, or tacos, use a 50:50 mixture of beef and TSP or, if you find the flavor pleasing, just use TSP in place of beef. Because TSP is so low in moisture, it has a very long shelf-life. It will stay fresh in tightly covered containers at room temperature for several months. Once rehydrated, though, it must be refrigerated and used within a few days.

Vegetarian TSP and Mushroom Stroganoff

1   large onion, chopped
4   tablespoons olive oil, plus
        1 teaspoon sweet butter
4   large Portobello mushrooms,
        cleaned and sliced
1½ cups vegetable stock
½   cup TSP, rehydrated with
        ¾ cup plus 1 teaspoon hot
        water

2   tablespoons flour
1   cup fat-free sour cream
    Yolk-free broad noodles,
        cooked
    Chopped fresh parsley

Sauté the onions in olive oil until translucent. Add the mushrooms and cook, stirring frequently, until soft. Add the vegetable stock and TSP. Stir the flour into the sour cream, then add it slowly to the mushroom/TSP/stock, stirring constantly to make a smooth, creamy sauce. Serve over noodles, garnished with chopped fresh parsley.

Yield: 4 servings

Soy protein: 3 g per serving
Soy isoflavones: variable

TSP Sloppy Joes

4   Kaiser rolls
1   cup rehydrated TSP

1   can sloppy joe sauce
4   slices onion

Slice the rolls and warm them in the oven while heating the TSP in the sloppy joe sauce. Remove the rolls from the oven, put 1 slice of onion on the bottom half of each roll, add the sloppy joe mixture, and top with the second half of the roll.

Yield: 4 sandwiches

Soy protein: 4 g per sandwich
Soy isoflavones: variable

SOY FLOUR

Soy flour is a fine, protein-rich powder that is produced by grinding roasted soybeans. It comes in two versions, full-fat ("natural") soy flour and fat-free soy flour (flour from which the oils are removed during processing).

Soy flours are most commonly found in processed foods such as candies, baked goods, pasta, and frozen desserts, as well as in prepared meat products such as meatloaves. But they also work well in home cooking and baking, in practically every dish ordinarily made with wheat flours.

For example, you can use soy flour to thicken gravies and sauces. Or you can use it as "breading" (coating) for fried foods. You can also use soy flour in baked goods, but because it does not contain gluten (the protein in wheat flour that traps air and enables bread to rise), you can't use it alone in cakes and breads.

Table 7-1 lists simple rules from the United Soybean Board for soy flour substitution.

Soy flours add a pleasant nutty flavor to baked goods. You can intensify the flavor by lightly toasting the flour; just heat it for several minutes in a dry skillet, stirring constantly to prevent burning. Breads and cakes made with soy flour tend to brown more quickly than those made with wheat flour alone. To compensate, you may have to lower the baking temperature a bit or slightly shorten the baking time. Don't be afraid to experiment. The result will be worth the trouble. By the way, to protect your soy flours from rancidity, store them in the refrigerator or freezer.

Here's a culinary curiosity. Because soy flour is a humectant (an ingredient that holds moisture), you can use it, in limited quantities,

Table 7-1 Simple Rules of Soy Flour Substitution

---

1. In a yeast bread, you may substitute soy flour for up to 15% of the wheat flour in the recipe.
2. In a no-yeast baked product, such as a cake, you may substitute soy flour for up to 25% of the wheat flour in the recipe.
3. To measure out soy flour that is equal to 15% of 1 cup of flour, put 2 tablespoons of soy flour in a 1-cup measuring cup and then fill the cup with the flour that is suggested for the recipe.

---

as a cholesterol-free egg substitute in baking. One tablespoon of soy flour plus 1 tablespoon water will replace 1 egg in a 2-egg (or more) recipe.

Basic Soy Flour Bread (*)

2 cups milk	½ cup warm water (about
⅔ cup brown sugar, packed	120 degrees)
⅓ cup margarine	1 egg, beaten
2 cups soy flour	1 tablespoon salt
1 tablespoon dry active yeast	4½ to 5 cups all-purpose flour

Heat the milk gently. Stir in the brown sugar, margarine, and soy flour. Beat until smooth, then remove from the stove and cool.

Dissolve the yeast in the warm water. Add the dissolved yeast, egg, salt, and 4½ cups of all-purpose flour to the soy flour/milk mixture. Mix well.

Turn it out onto a lightly floured surface and knead until the dough is smooth and elastic, about 10 minutes. Add the remaining all-purpose flour as needed to make a dough that handles well and does not stick to your fingers.

Roll the dough into a ball and put it in the greased bowl. Turn it once to coat the top of the dough ball, cover it, and set it aside to rise overnight (customarily 8 to 10 hours) to accommodate the soy flour, which does not rise like wheat flours, at room temperature.

Grease two 9 x 5-inch loaf pans and set them aside. Punch down the dough, and knead it until smooth. Divide it in half, shape it into two loaves, and place them in loaf pans. Cover and let them rise in a warm place for 1 to 2 hours or until they are double in size.

Preheat the oven to 375 degrees. Bake the loaves for 45 minutes. If the loaves begin to brown too quickly, cover them loosely with aluminum foil until they are completely baked.

Yield: 2 loaves

Soy protein: 5 g in 1 slice of a 16-slice loaf made with full-fat soy flour; 7 g in 1 slice of a 16-slice loaf made with defatted soy flour
Soy isoflavones: 6.25 in 1 slice of a 16-slice loaf

Soy Flour Pie Crust (*)

¾ cup unsifted flour   ⅓ cup shortening
¾ cup soy flour   4   to 5 tablespoons cold water
½ teaspoon salt

Preheat the oven to 400 degrees. Mix the flours and salt thoroughly. Cut the shortening into the flour mixture, using a pastry cutter or a fork, until the mixture is crumbly.

Add the water, a tablespoon at a time, while mixing gently. The dough should be just moist enough to cling together when pressed.

Shape the dough into two balls. Roll each ball out on a lightly floured surface until the dough is at least one inch wider all around than the pie pan in which you plan to use it. Fold each circle of dough in half and lift it into the pie pan; unfold and fit the dough gently to the pan. Trim the edges and shape the pastry rim as desired. Prick the bottom and sides with a fork. Bake 12 to 15 minutes, until golden brown.

Yield: Two 9-inch pie crusts

Soy protein: 60 g in one pie crust made with full-fat soy flour; 81 g in one pie crust made with defatted soy flour
Soy isoflavones: 75 mg per pie crust

Soy Milk

Soy milk is a thick white liquid made from soy flour (ground soybeans) and water. Plain soy milk is a cholesterol-free creamy beverage. Fat-free soy milk is also cholesterol-free, but because it has no fat, it tastes "skinnier" and less creamy than regular soy milk, just as fat-free skim cow's milk tastes thinner and less creamy than full-fat whole milk.

You can buy liquid soy milk in aseptic packages that store well at room temperature. Once opened, however, they must be refrigerated. Like regular milk, soy milk is also available as an instant powder that should be stored in the refrigerator or freezer. Both liquid soy milk and powdered soy milk come plain or flavored. Judging by the selection on the shelf at my favorite health food stores, the most popular flavored soy milk is vanilla.

You can use soy milk any way you use cow's milk or cream: on cereal; in coffee; in cakes, custards, and pancakes; or as a base for cream soups. Use powdered soy milk as a base for a quick meal.

Home-Made Soy Milk (*)

3 cups water
1 cup full-fat soy flour or 1 cup fat-free flour

Bring the water to a full boil. Pour the soy flour slowly into the water, stirring constantly to prevent lumps. Reduce the heat and simmer the mixture for about 20 minutes, stirring from time to time to keep the liquid smooth. While the milk is cooking, line a colander with cheesecloth. Then strain the cooked milk through the colander into a large bowl or glass container. Refrigerate, and use within a few days.

Yield: 4 cups

Soy protein: 20 g per cup of milk made with full-fat soy flour; 27 g in 1 cup of milk made with defatted soy flour
Soy isoflavones: 25 mg per cup of milk

Creamy Tomato Soup (+)

1	medium onion, diced	½	teaspoon salt
2	teaspoons soy oil	½	teaspoon ground white
1	large tomato, peeled,		pepper
	seeded, and diced	1	cup soy milk
½	teaspoon chopped garlic	10½	ounces silken tofu
1	teaspoon fresh basil,		
	chopped		

Sauté the onion with the oil in a saucepan for 3 minutes or until transparent. Add the tomato and garlic, continuing to sauté for 2 to 3 minutes. Add the basil, salt, and pepper. Blend in the soy milk. Cook, stirring constantly, for 1 minute. Remove it from the heat and cool it briefly. Transfer the soup to the food processor, add the tofu, and blend it until smooth. Serve hot or chilled.

Yield: 4 servings

Soy protein: 5 g per serving of soup made with full-fat soy milk; 7 g per serving of soup made with defatted soy flour
Soy isoflavones: 6 mg per cup of soup

"Your Choice" Vegetable Cream Soup

6 medium carrots, sliced; or
     1 (10-ounce) package
     frozen peas; or 5 medium
     tomatoes, peeled, seeded,
     and sliced; or 10 ounces
     fresh white mushrooms,
     cleaned and sliced; or
     1 cup frozen corn kernels
2 cups vegetable or chicken
     stock

1 small onion, chopped (omit
     for onion soup)
1 teaspoon curry powder
1 teaspoon cumin
½ cup soy milk
     Parsley
     Salt to taste

Choose the vegetable you prefer. Add the vegetable to the stock, chopped onion, curry, and cumin in saucepan. Simmer them over low heat until the vegetables are soft, then pour the mixture into a blender and puree. Return mixture to the saucepan, add the soy milk, and heat. Pour it into soup bowls and garnish with parsley, salt to taste.

Yield: 4 servings

Soy protein: 2.5 g per serving of soup made with full-fat soy milk; 3.5 g per serving of soup made with defatted soy flour
Soy isoflavones: 3 mg per cup of soup

SOY SAUCES

Soy sauce is the liquid extracted from aged, fermented soybeans or from a mixture of aged, fermented soybeans and wheat. Tamari is a soy sauce made from plain beans. Teriyaki is a soy sauce made from plain beans, then thickened with sugar, and seasoned with vinegar and other spices. Shoyu is a soy sauce made from soybeans and wheat.

Soy sauces are used as a salty condiment, as a flavor accent in dipping sauces for dumplings or other foods, and as marinades. In your kitchen, they can be stored at room temperature or refrigerated.

Soy Dipping Sauce

½ cup tamari
½ teaspoon hot sesame oil
¼ teaspoon sliced green onions

Mix the ingredients and use the sauce for dipping dumplings, tempura (deep-fried) vegetables, and so forth.

Yield: ½ cup

Soy protein: Soy sauces are not a source of soy protein.
Soy isoflavones: Soy sauces are not a source of isoflavones.

Teriyaki Lamb Chops or Chicken Leg Quarters

8   baby lamp chops or 8 chicken leg quarters
½   cup teriyaki sauce

Arrange the lamb chops or chicken in a baking dish. Pour the teriyaki sauce over the chops, cover them, and refrigerate for about 1 hour. Turn the chops over in the dish to marinate the other side and return them to refrigerate for another hour.

Prepare the chops by broiling them until they are done or by grilling them on a barbecue.

Yield: 4 servings

Soy protein: Soy sauces are not a source of soy protein.
Soy isoflavones: Soy sauces are not a source of isoflavones.

SOYBEAN OIL

Two things set the soybean apart from other beans. The first is its protein, complete with all the amino acids that are essential for human health. The second is its high fat content. More than 40% of the calories in soybeans come from its heart-healthy, cholesterol-free oil, low in saturated fats and high in poly- and monounsaturates.

You can use soybean oil in any recipe calling for a vegetable oil. Unlike other oils such as peanut oil and olive oil, soybean oil has no distinctive flavor of its own to mask or change the flavor of food. Safety-conscious cooks will be interested to hear that soybean oil's smoking point (the temperature at which it begins to smoke and burn) is higher than the smoking point for butter, 440 degrees for soybean oil versus 375 degrees for butter. Unfortunately, soybean oil is a poor choice for deep frying because it foams when heated.

Italian Salad Dressing (+)

5 tablespoons red wine vinegar	½ teaspoon salt
¼ cup water	⅛ teaspoon ground black pepper
¼ cup soybean oil	
1 teaspoon Italian seasoning (basil, oregano, thyme)	

Combine all of the ingredients in a jar and shake well.

Yield: About ½ cup

Soy protein: Soybean oil is not a source of soy protein.
Soy isoflavones: Soybean oil is not a source of isoflavones.

MISO

Miso is a salty condiment that is made by mixing cooked soybeans with salt and a fermenting agent called koji. You can usually find miso at Asian food stores, where it is sold either as a paste or as a dehydrated product. Paste or dehydrated, miso ranges in color from creamy to dark brown; the darker the color, the stronger the flavor.

Miso paste stays fresh for about six months, preferably in the refrigerator. Dehydrated miso should be stored in a cool, dry place. Is there white mold growing on your miso? This is common with fermented foods and, says the United Soybean Board, is harmless. Just scrape it off.

Use miso to flavor soups, sauces, dressings, and marinades. You can substitute miso for Worcestershire sauce or salt, adding protein along with flavor. Miso soup, regarded as an appetizer in the United States, is the quintessential breakfast dish in Japan.

Miso Soup (*)

3 cups water	1 cup cooked Japanese ramen
1 small onion, sliced	noodles
3 heaping tablespoons miso	

Bring the water to a simmer and add the onion. Cook until the onion is tender. Take a small amount of water from the pot and mix it with the miso to make a smooth paste. Add the miso paste to the water and onion. Simmer for 10 minutes. Add the cooked noodles and simmer gently just long enough to heat through. Serve immediately.

Yield: 4 servings

Soy protein: 1.5 g per serving
Soy isoflavones: 15 mg per serving

Miso Salad Dressing (*)

2 tablespoons miso
⅓ cup water
¼ cup soy oil

3 tablespoons rice vinegar
1 tablespoon honey
¼ tablespoon dry mustard

Stir the miso and water together into a smooth paste. Add the remaining ingredients and stir until blended. Serve over a salad or vegetables.

Yield: 1 cup

Soy protein: 4 g per cup
Soy isoflavones: 13 mg per cup

Miso Barbecue Sauce (*)

1 tablespoon miso
¼ cup water
1 tablespoon toasted sesame
   seeds
3 green onions, chopped

4 cloves garlic, minced
2 tablespoons sesame oil
2 tablespoons maple syrup
2 tablespoons sherry
⅛ tablespoon ground pepper

Blend miso and water. Add the remaining ingredients and mix well. Refrigerate until ready to use.

Yield: 1 cup sauce

Soy protein: 2 g per cup
Soy isoflavone: 7 mg per cup

Miso Sauce for Vegetables or Rice

1   tablespoon miso
1   tablespoon white wine

1   tablespoon maple syrup
1   tablespoon minced onion

Mix all of the ingredients thoroughly. Use this as a dressing for hot vegetables, including potatoes, or thin it with a little water and use it as a sauce for rice.

Yield: ⅓ cup sauce

Soy protein: .7 g per ⅓ cup
Soy isoflavones: 2.3 mg per ⅓ cup

Appendix A

Shopping for Soy Through the Mail

Hate to drag a shopping cart around the supermarket aisles? Well, you're in luck. Many mail-order food companies stock a variety of soy products, from the bean to prepared meals. As a bonus, you get a catalog with lots of other yummy foodstuffs, cookbooks, health books, herbals, cosmetics, and other goodies, and the only thing you have to exercise is your dialing finger!

Community Mill & Bean Inc.
267 Route 89 South
Savannah, NY 13146
Telephone: (315) 365-2664
Fax: (315) 365-2690
Soy products: soybeans, soy flour.

Devansoy Farms Inc.
P.O. Box 885
Carroll, IA 51401
Telephone: (712) 792-9665
Fax: (712) 792-2712
Soy products: soy flour, soy milk drinks, soy milk powders, tofu powder.

Dixie USA, Inc.
P.O. Box 55549
Houston, TX 77255
Telephone: (713) 688-4993
Fax: (800) 688-2507
Website: www.dixieusa.com/DDC.html
Soy products: baked goods (with soy flour); cereals; dairy substitutes (milk, creamer, yogurt); entrée mixes and kits (meatloaf, chicken and dumplings,

pizza, spaghetti and meat sauce, burritos, lasagna, and casseroles); flours; meat substitute mixes (burgers, tacos, chili, "chicken"); meat substitutes (chunks, strips, ground); nutrient bars. Also: cookbooks, kitchenware, condiments, substitutes (fats, eggs, sweeteners).

Ener-G Foods
5960 1st Avenue South
P.O. Box 84487
Seattle, WA 96124-5787
Telephone: (800) 331-5222
Fax: (206) 764-3398
Soy products: soy milk (instant). Also: gluten-free and wheat-free bake mixes, baked goods, cereals, gelatin desserts, pasta, soup mixes, and cookbooks (gluten-free recipes).

Gold Mine Natural Food Company
3419 Hancock Street
San Diego, CA 92110-4307
Telephone: (800) 475-3663
Soy products: miso (barley, rice, grain-free); natto soybeans (yellow, black); soy sauces (shoyu and tamari); soy meat substitute; soy milks. Also: personal care products, household products, kitchen tools, cookbooks, health books.

Grandma Beth's Cookies
1221 Toluca
Alliance, NE 69301
Telephone: (308) 762-8433
Website: www.avn.net/grandmabeths
Soy products: tofu, tofu products (including cookies).
Innovations Unlimited
5700 Loch Woode Court
Holt, MI 48842
Telephone: (517) 694-5348
Soy products: soynut butter, soynuts.

Lee Seed Farm
2242 Highway 182
Inwood, IA 51240
Telephone: (712) 753-4403
Soy products: soynuts, whole soybeans.

The Mail Order Catalog
Box 180
Summertown, TN 38483
Telephone: (800) 695-2241
E-mail: catalog@usit.net
Website: www.healthy-eating.com
Soy products: soy milk powder (low-fat), soy milk creamer (instant), soynut butter, soynuts (roasted), soy protein isolate, tempeh starter, texturized vegetable protein, tofu breading mixes. Also: cookbooks, herbal products.

Natural Lifestyle
16 Lookout Drive
Asheville, NC 28804-3330
Telephone: (800) 752-2775; (704) 242-9606
Fax: (704) 252-3386
E-mail: nicat@natural-lifestyle.com
Website: www.natural-lifestyle.com
Soy products: miso, miso soup, natto miso, soy-based mayonnaise substitute, soy milks and beverages, soy sauces (shoyu, tamari) tofus, tofu salad dressings. Also: personal health care products, herbal products, cosmetics, kitchen and laundry products, kitchenware, linens and natural fiber clothing, cookbooks, health books, video filters.

Phipps Country
P.O. Box 349
Pescadero, CA 94060
Telephone: (800) 279-0889; (650) 879-0787
Fax: (650) 879-1622
Soy products: soybeans (dried), soy flour (defatted). Also: herbs and spices, beans, grains, baking mixes, honeys, beeswax products.

Something Better Natural Foods
614 Capital Avenue N.E.
Battle Creek, MI 49017
Telephone: (616) 965-1199
Fax: (616) 965-8500
Soy products: soy milk beverages, soy milk powders, soy flour, soybeans, soy nuts, texturized soy protein.

South River Miso Company
888 Shelburne Falls Road
Conway, MA 01341
Telephone: (413) 369-4057
Fax: (413) 369-4299
Soy products: miso.

Weide Nutrition Group
1960 South 4250 West
Salt Lake City, UT 84104
Telephone: (801) 975-5000
Soy products: soy milk beverages.

Wellspring Natural Food Company
P.O. Box 2473
Amherst, MA 01004
Telephone: (800) 576-5301; (413) 323-7809
Fax: (413) 323-7993
E-mail: wspring@javanet.com
Soy products: miso, soybeans (dried), soy milks, soy sauces (shoyu). Also: body care products, household supplies, kitchenware, audio and video tapes, cookbooks.

Appendix B

Directory of Soy Manufacturers

No matter how many mail-order firms open for business, eventually we have to make the trip to the supermarket. The good news is that these days even small markets seem to carry a variety of brand name soy food products from (literally) "soup to nuts."

Got a question about one of these products? Get your answer by using the following list of selected companies from the U.S. 1997 Soyfoods Directory, published by the Indiana Soybean Development Council. To obtain your own copy of this useful booklet, which includes regional companies as well as the national organizations listed here, call (800) 301-3153. (P.S. The brand names listed below are trademarked.)

ADM (Archer Daniels Midland)
4666 Faries Parkway
Decatur, IL 62525
Telephone: (217) 424-2593
Fax: (217) 362-3959
Brand name soy products: Harvest Burgers, Nutrisoy.

Agronico
RR1, P.O. Box 55
Le Center, MN 56057
Telephone: (612) 357-4474
Fax: (612) 357-6388
Brand name soy products: Soja (soy beverages).
Amberwave Foods
625 Allegheny Avenue
Oakmont, PA 15139
Telephone: (412) 828-3152
Brand name soy products: Soydance Pizza.

American Natural Snacks
P.O. Box 167
St. Augustine, FL 32085
Telephone: (904) 825-2039
Brand name soy products: Soya Kass (cheese).

Arrowhead Mills
110 South Lawton
P.O. Box 2059
Hereford, TX 79045
Telephone: (806) 364-0730
Fax: (806) 364-8242
Brand name soy products:Arrowhead Mills Certified Organically Grown Soybean Flour, Arrowhead Mills Organically Grown Dry Soybeans.

Baycliff Company
242 East 72 Street
New York, NY 10021-4574
Telephone: (212) 772-6078
Brand name soy products: Sushi Chef (soy sauces, salad dressings).

Boca Burger Company
1660 N. E. 12th Terrace
Fort Lauderdale, FL 33305
Telephone: (954) 524-1977
Fax: (954) 524-4653
Website: www.gate.net/-BocaBurg
Brand name soy products: Boca Burgers, Chef Max's Favorite, Vegan Original.
Carnation Alsoy
800 N. Brand Boulevard
Glendale, CA 91203
Telephone: (800) 543-3112
Brand name soy products: Carnation Alsoy (infant formulas).

Cemac Foods Corporation
1821 East Sedgley Avenue
Philadelphia, PA 19124
Telephone: (215) 28807440
Fax: (215) 533-8993
Brand name soy products: NU-TOFU (cheese).

Champlain Valley Milling Corp.
P.O. Box 454
West Port, NY 12993-0454
Telephone: (516) 962-4711
Brand name soy products: Champlain Valley Milling Soy Flour.

Clements Foods Company
6601 N. Harvey Place
Okalahoma City, OK 73116
Telephone: (405) 842-3308
Brand name products: Garden Club Soy Sauce.

Colonel Sanchez Food
P.O. Box 5848
Santa Monica, CA 90940
Telephone: (310) 313-6769
Fax: (213) 732-2271
Brand name soy products: Red Chili Tofu Tamale.

Columbus Foods Company
800 N. Albany Avenue
Chicago, IL 60622
Telephone: (312) 265-6500
Fax: (312) 265-6985
Brand name soy products: Mike Soybean Oil, Sun Soybean Oil.
Eden Foods Inc.
701 Tecumseh Road
Clinton, MI 49236
Telephone: (517) 456-7424
Fax: (517) 456-7025
Brand name soy products: Edensoy (soy beverages), Edensoy Extra (soy beverages), Eden Blend (soy/rice beverages), Eden (miso, soy sauces, dried tofu).

Ener-G Foods Inc.
5960 1st Avenue
S. Seattle, WA 98108
Telephone: (800) 331-5222
Fax: (206) 764-3398
Brand name soy products: Soyquick (soy beverage).

Fantastic Foods Inc.
1250 N. McDowell Boulevard
Petaluma, CA 94954
Telephone: (707) 778-7801
Fax: (707) 778-6208
Brand name soy products: Fantastic Foods (meat alternatives, miso, TSP, tofu and tofu products).

Felbro Food Products Inc.
5700 W. Adams Boulevard
Los Angeles, CA 90016
Telephone: (213) 936-5266
Fax: (213) 936-5946
Brand name soy products: Felbro (salad dressings, soy sauces).

Gateway Food Products Company
1728 N. Main Street
Dupo, IL 62239
Telephone: (314) 231-9932
Fax: (618) 286-3444
Brand name soy products: Gateway Soy Brand Shortening.

Great Eastern Sun Inc.
92 McIntosh Road
Asheville, NC 28800
Telephone: (704) 665-7790
Fax: (704) 667-8051
Brand name soy products: Emperor's Kitchen (soy sauces), MasterMiso (miso).

Hartz Jacob Seed Company
Box 946
Stuttgart, AR 72160
Telephone: (501) 673-8565
Brand name soy products: Hartz Jacob Natto, Hartz Jacob soybeans.

Harvest Direct
P.O. Box 988
Knoxville, TN 37901-0988
Telephone: (423) 523-2304
Fax: (423) 523-3372
E-mail: harvest@slip.net
Brand name soy products: Harvest Direct Protein (burger mixes).

Hormel Foods Corporation
P.O. Box 800
Austin, MN 55912-0800
Telephone: (507) 437-5611
Brand name soy products: House of Tsang (soy sauces).

House Foods America Corp.
526 Stanford Avenue
Los Angeles, CA 90013-2123
Telephone: (213) 624-3615
Brand name soy products: Hinoichi (tofu and tofu products).
Houston Calco Inc.
2400 Dallas Street
Houston, TX 77003
Telephone: (713) 236-8668
Fax: (713) 236-1920
E-mail: kent@hypercon.com
Brand name soy products: ToFu, Soy Bean Milk (drinks, powders).

Hybco, U.S.A.
333 Mission Road
Los Angeles, CA 90033
Telephone: (213) 269-3111
Fax: (213) 269-3130
Brand name soy products: Certified Kosher Plant (soy oil and shortenings).

Island Spring Inc.
P.O. Box 747
Vashon, WA 98070
Telephone: (206) 463-9648
Fax: (206) 463-5670
Brand name soy products: Island Spring (soy milk, tofu burgers, tofu, tofu products).

Jaclyn's Food Products Inc.
P.O. Box 1314
Cherry Hill, NJ 08034
Telephone: (609) 354-2267
Fax: (609) 354-8335
Website: www.hlthmall.com.healthmall/jaclyns/
Brand name soy products: Jaclyn's Cheese Pizza, Fat Free (with soy cheese).

Kikkoman Foods Inc.
Highway 14 & Six Corners Road
Walworth, WI 53184
Telephone: (414) 275-6181
Fax: (414) 275-9452
Brand name soy products: Kikkoman (soy sauces, basting products, glazes).
LaChoy Food Products
901 Stryker Street
Archbold, OH 43502
Telephone: (714) 680- 1000
Brand name soy products: LaChoy (soy sauce).

Legume Inc.
112 Main Road
Montville, NJ 07045-9777
Telephone: (712) 753-4403
Brand name soy products: Barat Tofu Chocolate, Legume Frozen
Entrees, Legume Healthy Vegetarian Meals in a Can.

Lightlife Foods
P.O. Box 870
Greenfield, MA 01302
Telephone: (413) 774-6001
Fax: (413) 772-2682
Brand name soy products: Smart Dogs, Tofu Pups, Lean Links, Breakfast Fakin
Bacon, Smart Deli Slices, Classic Sloppy J's Chia Chili, Lightburgers, Wonder-
dogs, Gimme Lean, Vegetarian Request (frozen entrees and dinners).

Lucas Meyer Inc.
765 E. Pythian Avenue
P.O. Box 3218
Decatur, IL 62524
Telephone: (800) SOY-3660
Fax: (217) 877-5046
Brand name soy products: Epikuron, Emulpur, Nurupan, Soyapan.

Lumen Foods, Herbologics Inc.
409 Scott Street
Lake Charles, LA 70601
Telephone: (318) 438-6748
Fax: (318) 436-1769
Brand name soy products: Heartline Meatless Entrees, Heartline Meatless
Meats, Cajun Jerky, Stonewall's Jerquee, Heaven on Earth Soymilk Replacer.

Mandarin Soy Sauce Inc.
419 North Street
Middletown, NY 10940
Telephone: (914) 343-1505
Fax: (914) 343-0731
Brand name soy products: Wanjashan (soy sauces).

Marburger Foods
P.O. Box 387
Peru, IN 46970
Telephone: (317) 473-3086
Fax: (317) 473-8554
Brand name soy products: Bacon Bits.

Miyako Oriental Foods Inc.
4287 Puente Avenue
Baldwin Park, CA 91706
Telephone: (818) 962-9633
Fax: (818) 814-4569
Brand name soy products: Cold Mountain Miso, Yamajirushi Miso.

Morinaga Nutritional Foods Inc.
2050 West 190th Street
Suite 110
Torrance, CA 90504
Telephone: (310) 787-0200; (800) NOW-TOFU
Fax: (310) 787-2727
Brand name soy products: Mori-Nu (tofus).

Nasoya Foods
23 Jytek Drive
Leominster, MA 01453
Telephone: (508) 537-0713
Fax: (508) 537-9790
Brand name soy products: Nayonaise (soy-based dressing), New Menu Vegi/Burger, New Menu Vegi/Dog, New Menu Tofu/Mate.
Natural Way Mills Inc.
Route 2, Box 37
Middle River, MN 56737
Telephone: (218) 222-3677
Fax: (218) 222-3408
Brand name soy products: Nature's Hilights Soy Cheese Pizza (see next entry), Nature's Hilights Soy Cheese Tostadas (see next entry).

Nature's Hilights
1604 West 5th Street
P.O. Box 3526
Chico, CA, 95927
Telephone: (800) 313-6454
Brand name soy products: Nature's Hilights Soy Cheeses.

Northern Soy, SoyBoy
545 West Avenue
Rochester, NY 14611
Telephone: (716) 235-8970
Fax: (716) 235-3753
Brand name soy products: SoyBoy Tempeh, SoyBoy Tofu (and tofu products), SoyBoy NOT DOGS and Leaner Weiners, Okaru Courage Burger, Okaru Ravioli.

Nutritious Foods
P.O. Box 1606
St. Louis, MO 63188
Telephone: (800) 446-3350
Brand name soy products: Take Care (isolated soy protein beverage powders).

P. J. Lisac & Associates Inc.
9001 S. E. Lawnfield Road
Clackamas, OR 97015
Telephone: (503) 652-1988
Fax: (503) 686-6509
Brand name soy products: Lisanetti Soy-Satin (soy cheese).

Pacific Foods of Oregon Inc.
19480 SW 97th Avenue
Tualatin, OR 97062
Telephone: (503) 692-9666
Fax: (503) 692-9610
Brand name soy products: Pacific Brands (soy milk drinks, tofu, tofu products).

PEDCO
270 7th Street
Wheeling, IL 60090
Telephone: (647) 541-5513
Brand name soy products: DeWeese Nutty Soynuts, DeWeese Nutty Soys.

Perk-Up
4 Division Street
Tarrytown, NY 10591
Telephone: (914) 631-5595
Fax: (914) 631-0854
Brand name soy products: Panda-Chinese and American Soy Sauce.

PMS Foods Inc.
2701 East 11th Street
P.O. Box 1099
Hutchinson, KS 67504-1099
Telephone: (316) 663-5711
Fax: (316) 663-7195
E-mail: Dpark@southwind.net
Brand name soy products: Ultra Soy Textured Soy Flour (meat alternatives).

Proctor & Gamble Company
6071 Center Hill Road
Cincinnati, OH 45224
Brand name soy products: Crisco.

Protein Technologies International
Checkerboard Square
St. Louis, MO 63132
Telephone: (314) 982-3692
Brand name soy products: Supro and Take Care (soy protein isolates, soybean meal, soy flakes, soy flour, oil, and shortenings).

Quong Hop & Company
161 Beacon Street
S. San Francisco, CA 94080
Telephone: (415) 761-2022
Fax: (415) 952-3329
Brand name soy products: Soy Deli, Quong Hop, Gold Mountain, Pacific, Soy Fresh (soymilk drinks, tempeh, tofu, and tofu products).

Rich Products Corporation
1150 Niagara Street
P.O. Box 246
Buffalo, NY 14240
Telephone: (716) 878-8000
Fax: (716) 878-8238
Brand name soy products: Rich (isolated soy protein, frozen desserts, protein concentrates, whipped toppings, oil, and shortening).

Rosewood Products Inc.
738 Airport Boulevard
Ann Arbor, MI 48108
Telephone: (313) 665-2222
Fax: (313) 668-8430
Brand name soy products: China Rose, Rosewood Farms (meat alternatives, tofu, tempeh, soy milks, cheeses, fiber, drinks, frozen desserts).

Season's Harvest
52 Broadway
Somerville, MA 02145
Telephone: (617) 628-1182
Fax: (617) 628-1722
E-mail: ademar@braziltrade.com
Sharon's Finest
P.O. Box 5020
Santa Rosa, CA 95402-5020
Telephone: (707) 576-7050
Fax: (707) 545-7116
E-mail: richard@rella.com
Website: www.rella.com
Brand name soy products: TofuRella, TofuRella slices, VeganRella, Almond-Rella, Zero-FatRella, HempRella, Hempeh.

Simply Delicious Inc.
8411 Highway N.C. 86 N.
Cedar Grove, NC 27231
Telephone: (919) 732-5294
Brand name soy products: Simply Delicious Soy Gold (soy sauce).

Sno Pac Foods Inc.
379 S. Pine Street
Caledonia, MN 55921
Telephone: (507) 724-5281
Fax: (701) 642-4102
Brand name soy products: Sno Pac (whole soybeans).

Solnuts Inc.
711 Seventh Street
Hudson, IA 50643
Telephone: (319) 988-3221
Fax: (319) 988-4647
Brand name soy products: Solnut (soynuts, soy flour).

Sovex Foods Inc.
P.O. Box 2178
Collegedale, TN 37315
Telephone: (800) 227-2320
Fax: (615) 396-3402
Brand name soy products: Better Than Milk (soy milk).
Soyco Foods, Galaxy Foods Company
2441 Viscount Row
Orlando, FL 32809
Telephone: (800) 441-9419
Fax: (407) 855-7485
Brand name soy products: Lite & Less, Soyco, Soymage (cheese alternatives),
Garden Accents.

Soyfoods of America
1091 E. Hamilton Road
Duarte, CA 91010-2743
Telephone: (818) 358-3836
Brand name soy products: Furamna, Nature's Spring (tofu and tofu products).

Springfield Creamery
29440 Airport Road
Eugene, OR 97402
Telephone: (541) 689-2911
Fax: (541) 689-2915
Brand name soy products: Nancy's Cultured Soy Yogurt.

Sunlight Foods Inc.
3550 N. W. 112 Street
Miami, FL 33167
Telephone: (305) 688-5400
Fax: (305) 688-9903
Brand name soy products: Sunlight, Gold Label, Briar Hill (salad dressings,
soy sauces).

Sunrich
P.O. Box 128
101 Elevator Road
Hope, MN 56046
Telephone: (800) 342-6976
Fax: (507) 451-2910
Brand name soy products: SunRich Sweet Bean, SunRich Edamame, SunRich
Supreme Soymilk.

Sweet Earth Natural Foods
207 16th Street
Pacific Grove, CA 93950
Telephone: (408) 375-8673
Fax: (408) 375-3441
Brand name soy products: Sweet Earth (burgers), Savory Soy (burger).

Sycamore Creek Company, Inari Ltd.
200 State Street
Mason, MI 48854
Telephone: (517) 676-3826
Fax: (517) 676-6721
Brand name soy products: Nutty Nuggets, Morningstar Farms (soy butter), Natural Touch (soy butter), Sycamore Creek (soynut spread), Beanut Butter.

Tofutti Brands Inc.
50 Jackson Drive
Cranford, NJ 07016
Telephone: (908) 272-2400
Fax: (908) 272-9492
Brand name soy products: Tofutti (frozen dessert, cheese substitute, sour cream substitute, candy).

Tomanetti Foods Inc.
625 Allegheny Avenue
Oakmont, PA 15139
Telephone: (412) 828-3040
Fax: (412) 828-2282
Brand name soy products: Soydance Frozen Pizza.

Trophic International Inc.
464 West 3440 South
Salt Lake City, UT 84115-4228
Telephone: (801) 269-9960
Brand name soy products: Trophic's Best Tofu.
Tumaros/Homestyle Kitchens
5300 Santa Monica Boulevard
Los Angeles, CA 90029
Telephone: (213) 464-6317
Fax: (213) 464-7063
Brand name soy products: Homestyle Kitchen (soy cheese burritos, tofu enchiladas), BBQ Tofu.

Vitalite Foods
103 S. Westminster Street
P.O. Box 10
Waynesfield, OH 45896-0010
Telephone: (419) 568-8638
Brand name soy products: Cleveland Tofu, NuLinks (sausages), Vitalite Tofu,
Rippits Snacks (jerky).

Wan Ja Shan/Mandarin Soy Sauce
419 N. Street
Middletown, NY 10940-3603
Telephone: (914) 343-1505
Brand name soy products: Wan Ja Shan (soy sauces).

Westbrae Natural Foods
P.O. Box 48006
Gardena, CA 90248
Telephone: (310) 886-8200
Fax: (310) 886-8219
Brand name soy products: Black Soybean (miso, soy milk, tofu, tempeh, whole
soybeans, yuba).

White Wave Inc.
1990 N. 57th Court
Boulder, CO 80301
Telephone: (303) 443-3470
Fax: (303) 443-3952
Brand name soy products: White Wave (soy beverage, soy cheese, soy yogurt,
soy milk drinks, tempeh, tofu and tofu products, veggie franks).

Wis-Pak Foods
4700 N. 132nd Street
Butler, WI 53007
Telephone: (800) 558-2000
Fax: (414) 781-3538
Brand name soy products: Hearty Classics (burger, vegetarian chili, texturized
soy protein).

Worthington Foods Inc.
900 Proprietors Road
Worthington, OH 43085
Telephone: (614) 885-9511
Fax: (614) 885-2594
Brand name products: Morningstar Farms Grillers, Breakfast Strips; also: soy
milk drinks, soynut butter, tofu, and tofu products.

Appendix C

Directory of Soy Researchers Whose Studies Are Included in this Book

Herman Adlercreutz
Professor, Department of Clinical Chemistry
University of Helskini
Meilanhti Hospital
Helsinki, Finland 00290

James W. Anderson
Professor, Medical and Clinical Nutrition
University of Kentucky
Chief, Metabolic-Endocrine Section
VA Medical Center
2250 Leestown Road (111C)
Lexington, KY 40511-1093

Bahram H. Arjmandi
Assistant Professor, Human Nutrition and Dietetics
1919 West Taylor Street
Room 650
The University of Illinois at Chicago
Chicago, IL 60612

Mary Astuti
Lecturer, Faculty of Agriculture Technology
Gadjah Mada University
Balaksumur, Yogyakarta, Indonesia

Stephen Barnes
Associate Professor, Department of Biochemistry and Pharmacology
University of Alabama at Birmingham
Volker Hall
Room G010 UAB Station
Birmingham, AL 35294

Gregory L. Burke
Professor and Vice-Chairman
Department of Public Health Sciences
The Bowman Gray School of Medicine
Wake Forest University
Medical Center Boulevard
Winston-Salem, NC 27157-1063

Aedin Cassidy
Lecturer in Nutrition
Department of Nutrition
School of Biological Sciences
University of Surrey
Guildford, Surrey GU2 5XH
England

I. Catala
LEPSD
INRA
Jouy-en-Josas, France

John Anthony Eden
Associate Professor in Reproductive Endocrinology
University of New South Wales
Royal Hospital for Women
Barker Street (Locked Bag 2000)
Randwick, New South Wales
Australia 2031

Paolo Fanti
Assistant Professor
Division of Nephrology, Bone and Mineral Metabolism
University of Kentucky Medical Center
MN 642
800 Rose Street
Lexington, KY 40536

Maria Gabriella Gentile
Professor
Ospedale San Carlo Borromec
Servizio Di Dietollogia e Nutrizione Clinica
20153 Milano-via Pio Secondo, 3
Italy

William Helferich
Associate Professor
Department of Food Science and Human Nutrition
G. Malcolm Trout Food Science and Human Nutrition Building
Michigan State University
East Lansing, MI 48824-1224

Clifford H. G. Irvine
Professor Emeritus
AVSG
Lincoln University
Box 84
Canterbury, New Zealand

Elzbieta M. Kurowska
Research Associate
Department of Biochemistry
Centre for Human Nutrition
University of Western Ontario
London, Ontario N6A 5C1
Canada

Mindy Kurzer
Associate Professor
Department of Food Science and Nutrition
1334 Eckles Avenue
St. Paul, MN 53108-6099

Renee Lin
Professor of Medicine and Biochemistry/Molecular Biology
Indiana University School of Medicine
VA Medical Center
Research (151)
1481 West 10th Street
Indianapolis, IN 46202

Lee-Jane W. Lu
Associate Professor
Department Medicine and Community Health
The University of Texas Medical Branch
Galveston, TX 77555

Danielle F. McMichael-Phillips
Department of Epithelial Biology
Paterson Institute for Cancer Research
Christie Hospital NHS Trust
Wilmlow Road, Manchester M20 9BX
Manchester, England

Mark Messina
Nutrition Matters, Inc.
1543 Lincoln Street
Port Townsend, WA 98368

Alice Murkies
Consultant and Research Fellow
Jean Hailes Centre for Women
291 Clayton Road
Clayton, 3186 Australia

Karin Nilausen
Associate Professor
Department of Medical Anatomy
Section C
Panum Institute
University of Copenhagen
Blegdamsveg 3c
DK-2200
Copenhagen N, Denmark

Nicholas L. Petrakis
Professor and Chairman Emeritus of Preventive Medicine
    and Epidemiology
Department of Epidemiology and Biostatistics
Box 0560
MU-416 West
University of California, San Francisco
San Francisco, CA 94143-0560

John Potter
Program Head
Cancer Prevention Research Program
The Fred Hutchinson Cancer Research Centre
1124 Columbia Street
Seattle, WA 98104

Norbeta Schoene
Nutrient Requirements & Functions Laboratory
Beltsville Human Nutrition Research Center
United States Department of Agriculture Building 308
Room 114
Barc East
Beltsville, MD 20705-2350

Kenneth D. R. Setchell
Professor, Department of Pediatrics
Director, Clinical Mass Spectrometry Center
Children's Hospital and Medical Center
Elland and Bethesda Avenues
Cincinnati, OH 45229

Cesare R. Sirtori
Cattedra Di Farmacollogia Clinica
Universita Degli Studi De Milano
Instituto Di Scienza Farmacolohiche
20133 Milano, Via Balzaretti
Italy

Joanne Louise Slavin
Professor, Department of Food Science and Nutrition
University of Minnesota
1334 Eckles Avenue
St. Paul, MN 55108

William Wong
Professor, Department of Pediatrics USDA/ARS
Children's Nutrition Research Center
Stable Isotope Laboratory
1100 Bates Street, #7068
Houston, TX 77030-2600

Anna H. Wu
Associate Professor, Department of Preventive Medicine
1441 Eastlake Avenue
MS#44
University of Southern California
Los Angeles, CA 90033-0800

Shigeru Yamamoto
Professor, Department of Nutrition
Faculty of Medicine
University of Ryukyus
Okinawa 903-01, Japan

Sources

INTRODUCTION

Ackermann, A. S. E. *Popular Fallacies Explained and Corrected*, 3rd Edition (Philadelphia: Lippincott, 1924).

Fernie, W. T. *Meals Medicinal*. Bristol, England: John Wright & Co., 1905.

"School Buses to Try a Soybean Fuel," *New York Times* (December 6, 1997).

United Soybean Board. *Designed for Life*. St. Louis, n.d.

————*Soy: How a 5000-Year-Old Bean Is Making America Healthier*. St. Louis, n.d.

CHAPTER ONE: THE NUTRITIONAL WONDER BEAN

Calabrese article: www.life.ca/January 1997.

"Food Allergy Myths and Realities," *Food Insight Newsletter* (December 1997).

Gentile, Naria Gabriella, et al., "Soy Consumption and Renal Function in Patients with Nephrotic Syndrome: Clinical Effects and Potential Mechanism." Second International Symposium on the Role of Soy in Preventing and Treating Chronic Disease (Brussels, September 19, 1996).

Hasler, Claire. c-hasler@uiuc.edu (20 June 97).

Lowe, Carl. "The Iron Curd." *American Health* (April 1985).

"Mailbag." *Prevention Magazine* (December 1997).

Martinez, R. M., et al. "Soy Isoflavonoids Possess Biological Activities of Loop-Diuretics." Second International Symposium on the Role of

Soy in Preventing and Treating Chronic Disease (Brussels, September 19, 1996).

Menopause Online, www.infor@menopause-online.com.

Rinzler, Carol. *Nutrition for Dummies.* Foster City, Calif.: IDG Books, 1997.

United Soybean Board. *Designed for Life; Soy: How a 5000-Year-Old Bean Is Making Americans Healthier; Soybeans: Unlocking the Secret to Good Nutrition;* Soy Facts #10, *Soyfoods & Protein; Soyfood for Thought,* #9. St. Louis, n.d.

USDA. USDA Handbook No. 8-16 (Washington D.C., 1986).

Whitney, Eleanor Noss, Corrinne Balong Cataldo, and Sharon Rady Rolfes. *Understanding Normal and Clinical Nutrition.* Minneapolis/St. Paul: West Publishing Company, 1994.

CHAPTER TWO: SOMETHING SPECIAL IN THE BEAN

Barrett, J. "Phytoestrogens: Friends or Foes." *Environmental Health Perspectives,* 104 (1996):478–482.

Berrino, F. "A Randomized Trial to Prevent Hormonal Patterns at High Risk for Breast Cancer: The DIANA (Diet and Androgens) Project." Second International Symposium on the Role of Soy in Preventing and Treating Chronic Disease (Brussels, September 15–18, 1996).

Cole, Rebecca C., Jodi A. Flaws, and Trudy L. Bush. "Effects of Raloxifene in Postmenopausal Women," correspondence. *New England Journal of Medicine* (April 30, 1998).

Clemens, Roger A. "Health Implications of Dietary Phytoestrogens: A Food Industry Perspective." Institute of Food Technologists, 1997 Annual Meeting and Food Expo (Orlando, Florida, June 14–18, 1997).

Guillette, Louis J. "Ecoestrogens and Embryonic Abnormalities: Lessons from Wildlife." Institute of Food Technologists, 1997 Annual Meeting and Food Expo (June 14–18, 1997).

Hasler, Clarie. Re: "Chemistry of Soy." c-hasler@uiuc.edu (August 12, 1997).

Irvine, Clifford H. G., et al. "Isoflavone and Testosterone Extraction from Disposable Diapers: The New Zealand Experience." Second International Symposium on the Role of Soy in Preventing and Treating Chronic Disease (Brussels, September 15–18, 1996).

———"The Potential Adverse Effects of Soybean Phytoestrogens in Infants' Feeding." *New Zealand Medical Journal* 108 (1995): 208–109.

Makela, S. O., et al. "Phytoestrogens Are Partial Estrogen Agonists in the Adult Male Mouse." *Environmental Health Perspective* 103, supplement 7: 123–127.

Messina, Mark J., et al. *Nutrition and Cancer* 21 (1994):113.

Phipps, et al. "Effect of Flaxseed Ingestion on the Menstrual Cycle." *Journal of Clinical Endocrinology Metabolism* 77 (1993):1215– 1219.

"Phytoestrogens and Breast Cancer." Cornell University Program on Breast Cancer and Environmental Risk Factors in New York State, Fact Sheet #1 (November 1996).

"Phytoestrogens, Environmental Estrogens, and Other Hormones." Tulane and Xavier Universities, New Orleans, www.tmc.tulane. edu/cbr/ecme.

Raloff, Janet. "Plant Estrogens May Ward Off Breast Cancer." *Science News* (October 11, 1997).

Setchell, Kenneth D. "Overview of Isoflavone Structure, Metabolism, and Pharmokinetics." Second International Symposium on the Role of Soy in Preventing and Treating Chronic Disease (Brussels, September 15–18, 1996).

Slavin, Joanne L. "Effect of Wheat Bran on Metabolism of Chemopreventive Agents in Humans." Second International Symposium on the Role of Soy in Preventing and Treating Chronic Disease (Brussels, September 15–18, 1996).

Stob, Martin. "Estrogens in Foods." In *Toxicants Occurring Naturally in Foods,* Second Edition (Washington, D.C.: National Academy of Sciences, 1973).

United Soybean Board. Soy Facts #3, *Soy and Cancer*. St. Louis, n.d.

CHAPTER THREE: SOY AND YOUR HEART

American Heart Association. "Adding Progestins May Negate Heart Protection from Estrogen Replacement Therapy," Press Release (April 7, 1998).

———"1998 Heart and Stroke Statistical Update" (November 1997).

———. "Study Suggests Triglyceride Levels May Be Considered an Independent Risk Factor for Heart Attack in Some People." Press Release (March 23, 1998).

Anderson, James W., et al. "Meta-Analysis of the Effects of Soy Protein Intake on Serum Cholesterol" *New England Journal of Medicine* (August 3, 1995).

Anthony, M.D., et al. "Circulation 90" (supplement) l. (Abstr.). In Soy Facts #7, *Soyfoods and Isoflavones* (1994).

Astuti, Mary "The Role of Tempeh on Lipid Profile and Lipid Perox-idation." Second International Symposium on the Role of Soy in Preventing and Treating Chronic Disease (Brussels, September 15–18, 1996).

Catala, I., et al. "Use of Soy Proteins in Cholelithiasis Prevention." Second International Symposium on the Role of Soy in Preventing and Treating Chronic Disease (Brussels, September 15–18, 1996).

"Clinical News Digest." *US Pharmacist* (April 1998).

Gentile, Maria Gabriella, et al. "Soy Consumption and Renal Function in Patients with Nephrotic Syndrome: Clinical Effects and Potential Mechanism." Second International Symposium on the Role of Soy in Preventing and Treating Chronic Disease (Brussels, September 15–18, 1996).

Hadda, Ceri E. "Chick Beans." *American Health* (March 1986).

("Homocysteine?") *New York Times* (February 4, 1998).

Kurowska, Elzbieta M., et al. "Role of the Main Components of Whole Soybean Products, Soy Protein, and Soy Oil, in Reducing Hypercholesterolemia." Second International Symposium on the Role of Soy in Preventing and Treating Chronic Disease (Brussels, September 15–18, 1996).

Martinez, R. M., et al. "Soy Isoflavonoids Possess Biological Activities of Loop-Diuretics." Second International Symposium on the Role of Soy in Preventing and Treating Chronic Disease (Brussels, September 15–18, 1996).

"Menopause Online/Soyfoods": info@menopause-online.com.

Nilhausen, Karen, and Hanz Meinertz. "Variation in the Plasma Lipoprotein Response to Dietary Soy Protein in Normolipedemic Men." Second International Symposium on the Role of Soy in Preventing and Treating Chronic Disease (Brussels, September 15–18, 1996).

Rinzler, Carol Ann. *Complete Book of Food.* New York: Pharos, 1987.

Schoene, N. W., and C. A. Guidry. "Genistein Inhibits Reaction Oxygen Species (ROS) Formation During Activation of Rat Platelets in Whole Blood." Second International Symposium on the Role of Soy in Preventing and Treating Chronic Disease (Brussels, September 15–18, 1996).

Sitori, Cesare R. "Sorting Through Soy," letter. *Science News* (August 8, 1998).

Sirtori, Cesare R., et al. "Soy and Cholesterol Reduction: Clinical Experience and Molecular Mechanisms." Second International Symposium on the Role of Soy in Preventing and Treating Chronic Disease (Brussels, September 15–18, 1996).

Tierney, Lawrence N., et al. *Current Medical Diagnosis and Treatment*, 37th ed. Stamford, Conn.: Appleton & Lange, 1998.

United Soybean Board. *Soy: The Magic Bean*. St. Louis, n.d.

————. Soy Facts #5, *Soyfoods & Heart Disease*. St. Louis, n.d.

"Weight Loss Protects Heart." *US Pharmacist* (April 1998).

Wong, William W., et al. "Mechanisms for the Hypocholesterolemic Effect of Soy Protein in Normocholesterolemic and Hypercholesterolemic Men." Second International Symposium on the Role of Soy in Preventing and Treating Chronic Disease (Brussels, September 15–18, 1996).

Yamamoto, Shigeru, et al. "Anti-Cholesterolemic Effect of the Undigested Fraction of Soybean Protein," from the Dept. of Nutrition, Faculty of Medicine of the Ryukyus, Okinawa., Second International Symposium on the Role of Soy in Preventing and Treating Chronic Disease (Brussels, September 15–18, 1996).

CHAPTER FOUR: SOY, THE CANCER FIGHTER

American Cancer Society, "Cancer Facts and Figures, 1997 & 1998."

————. "Cancer Risk Report, 1996."

————. "Estrogen Replacement Therapy May Increase Women's Risk of Fatal Ovarian Cancer." Press Release (May 1, 1995).

American Heart Association, "Adding Progestins May Negate Heart Protection from Estrogen Replacement Therapy." Press Release (April 7, 1998).

Barnes, S. "A Double-Blind Clinical Trial of the Effects of Soy Protein on Risk Parameters for Prostate Cancer." Second International Symposium on the Role of Soy in Preventing and Treating Chronic Disease (Brussels, September 15–18, 1996).

Begley, Sharon, and Claudia Kalb. "One Man's Quest to Cure Cancer." *Newsweek* (May 18, 1998).

Berrino, F. "A Randomized Trial to Prevent Hormonal Patterns at High Risk for Breast Cancer: The DIANA (Diet and Androgens) Project." Second International Symposium on the Role of Soy in Preventing and Treating Chronic Disease (Brussels, September 15–18, 1996).

Cassidy, Aedin. "Hormonal Effects of Isoflavones on Humans." Second International Symposium on the Role of Soy in Preventing and Treating Chronic Disease (Brussels, September 15–18, 1996).

Elmore, Joann G., et al. "Ten Year Risk of False Positive Screening Mammograms and Clinical Breast Examinations." *New England Journal of Medicine* (April 16, 1998).

Environmental Health Perspective, 103, supplement 7: 123–127.

Goodman, Marc L., et al. "The Association of Dietary Phytoestrogens with the Risk for Endometrial Cancer." Second International Symposium on the Role of Soy in Preventing and Treating Chronic Disease (Brussels, September 15–18, 1996).

Hadda, Ceri. "Chick Beans." *American Health* (March 1986).

Hasler, Claire. "Chemistry of Soy." c-hasler@uiuc.edu (August 12, 1997).

———. c-hasler@uiuc.edu. (June 20, 1997).

Helferich, William G. "Paradoxical Effects of the Soy Phytoestrogen Genistein on the Growth of Human Breast Cancer Cells in Vitro and in Vivo." Institute of Food Technologists (1998).

Hempstock, J., et al. "Growth Inhibition of Human Prostatic Cell Lines by Phyto-Estrogens." Second International Symposium on the Role of Soy in Preventing and Treating Chronic Disease (Brussels, September 15–18, 1996).

Kennedy, Ann R. "The Bowman-Birk Inhibitor from Soybeans as an Anticancer Agent." Second International Symposium on the Role of Soy in Preventing and Treating Chronic Disease (Brussels, September 15–18, 1996).

Kurzer, Mindy S., et al. "Effects of Dietary Soy Isoflavones on Estrogen Action in Premenopausal Women." Second International Symposium on the Role of Soy in Preventing and Treating Chronic Disease (Brussels, September 15–18, 1996).

Lin, Renee C., and Ting-Kai Li, "Effects of Isoflavones on Alcohol Pharmokinetics and Alcohol Drinking Behavior." Second International Symposium on the Role of Soy in Preventing and Treating Chronic Disease (Brussels, September 15–18, 1996).

Lul, L. J. et al. "Reductions in Steroid and Gastrointestinal Hormone Levels in Men and Premenopausal Women with Soya Consumption for 1 Month." Second International Symposium on the Role of Soy in Preventing and Treating Chronic Disease (Brussels, September 15–18, 1996).

McMichael-Phillips, D. F., et al. "The Effects of Soy Supplementation on Epithelial Proliferation in the Normal Human Breast." Second International Symposium on the Role of Soy in Preventing and Treating Chronic Disease (Brussels, September 15–18, 1996).

"Menopause Online, Soy Foods." info@menopause-online.com.

"The Muddle over Screening Breast Cancer." *Medical World News* (May 9, 1988).

North American Menopause Society. "FAQS, 1997." www.menopause.org/home.htm.

Petrakis, Nicholas L., and Stephen Barnes (University of California S.F. and University of Alabama). "Stimulatory Effects of Soy Protein Isolate on Breast Fluid Secretion." Second International Symposium on the Role of Soy in Preventing and Treating Chronic Disease (Brussels, September 15–18, 1996).

Potter, John D. "Cancer Prevention: Food and Phytochemicals." Second International Symposium on the Role of Soy in Preventing and Treating Chronic Disease (Brussels, September 15–18, 1996).

Rao, A. V. "Anticarcinogenic Properties of Plant Saponins." Second International Symposium on the Role of Soy in Preventing and Treating Chronic Disease (Brussels, September 15–18, 1996).

Rinzler, Carol Ann. *Estrogen and Breast Cancer: A Warning to Women.* Alameda, Calif.: Hunter House, 1996.

"Risk of False Alarm from Mammogram is 50% over Decade." *New York Times* (April 16, 1998).

Sleicher, Rosemary, et al. "Genistein Inhibition of Prostate Cancer Cell Growth and Metastasis in Vivo." Second International Symposium on the Role of Soy in Preventing and Treating Chronic Disease (Brussels, September 15–18, 1996).

"Soy Intake May Reduce Risk of Uterine Cancer—New Cancer Research Study." Doctor's Guide/pslgroup.com/dg/36266 (1997).

"Soy Protein May Protect Against Breast Cancer. *Medical Sciences Bulletin* (November 1994) (Pharminfonet. home page).

Steele, Vernon E., et al. "Cancer Chemoprevention Agents Development Strategies for Genistein." *Journal of Nutrition* 125 (1995): 713S–716S.

United Soybean Board. Soy Facts #3, *Soy and Cancer.* St. Louis, n.d.

Wu, A. H. I., et al. "Tofu and Risk of Breast Cancer in Asian Americans." Second International Symposium on the Role of Soy in Preventing and Treating Chronic Disease (Brussels, September 15–18, 1996).

CHAPTER FIVE, BUILDING BETTER BONES WITH SOY

Arjmandi, B. H., et al. "A Soy Protein–Containing Diet Prevents Bone Loss due to Ovarian Hormone Deficiency." Second International Symposium on the Role of Soy in Preventing and Treating Chronic Disease (Brussels, September 15–18, 1996).

"Avoiding the Fracture Zone." *Nutrition Action Health Letter* (April 1998).

Blair, Harry C. "Action of Genistein and Other Tyrosine Kinase Inhibitors in Preventing Osteoporosis." Second International Symposium on the Role of Soy in Preventing and Treating Chronic Disease (Brussels, September 15–18, 1996).

Erdman, John W., et al. "Short-Term Effects of Soybean Isoflavones on Bone in Post-Menopausal Women." Second International Symposium on the Role of Soy in Preventing and Treating Chronic Disease (Brussels, September 15–18, 1996).

Fanti, Paolo, et al. "Systemic Administration of Genistein Partially Prevents Bone Loss in Ovarietomized Rats in a Non-Estrogen-Like Mechanism. Second International Symposium on the Role of Soy in Preventing and Treating Chronic Disease. (Brussels, September 15–18, 1996).

Fauci, Anthony S., et. al, ed., *Harrison's Principles of Internal Medicine*, 14th Ed. (New York: McGraw-Hill, 1998)

Getty, Vicky. "Soy Isoflavones and Bone Health" (11 August 1997), gettyv@efs.purdue.edu.

Hughes, Bess Dawson, et al. "Effect of Calcium and Vitamin K Supplementation on Bone Density in Men and Women 65 Years of Age or Older. *New England Journal of Medicine* (September 4, 1997).

Mayo Clinic. Mayo Clinic Health Letter, cited on (webmster @pslgroup.com).

Seppa, N. "Extra Calcium No Help for Lactating Women." *Science News* (August 23, 1997).

United Soybean Board. Soy Facts #2, *Soyfood and Bone Health*. St. Louis, n.d.

———. Soyfood for Thought #9, *Soyfoods Provide Many Essential Nutrients*. St. Louis, n.d.

USDA, Nationwide Food Consumption Survey, SURVEY, 1985. Report No. 85-4 (Hyattsville, Md.: USDA Nutrition Monitoring Division, Human Nutrition Information Service, 1987).

———. Vitamin K. U.S. Department of Agriculture Quarterly Report (July 1 to September 30, 1996).

CHAPTER SIX, HOT NEWS ABOUT HOT FLASHES

The Boston Women's Health Collective, *The New Our Bodies, Ourselves* (New York: Simon & Schuster, 1992).

Burke, Gregory L. "The Potential Use of a Dietary Soy Supplement as a Post-Menopausal Hormone Replacement Therapy." Second International Symposium on the Role of Soy in Preventing and Treating Chronic Disease (Brussels, September 15–18, 1996).

Duke, James. *Handbook of Medicinal Herbs* (Boca Raton, Fla.: CRC Press, 1988).

Dulais, F. S. I., et al. "Dietary Soy Supplementation Increases Vaginal Cytology Maturation Index and Bone Mineral Content in Postmenopausal Women." Second International Symposium on the Role of Soy in Preventing and Treating Chronic Disease (Brussels, September 15–18, 1996).

Eden, John Anthony, et al. "Hormonal Effects of Isoflavones." Second International Symposium on the Role of Soy in Preventing and Treating Chronic Disease (Brussels, September 15–18, 1996); personal correspondence, 1998.

Fackelmann, Kathleen. "Medicine for Menopause." *Science News* (June 20, 1998).

Hall, Celia. "Japanese Taste for Soy Protein Spares Them Hot Flashes." *The Electronic Press* (February 8, 1997).

"Menopause Online": info@menopause-online.com (dong quai, black cohosh).

Murkles, A. I., et al. "Dietary Flour Supplementation Decreases Post-Menopausal Hot Flushes: Effect of Soy and Wheat." Second International Symposium on the Role of Soy in Preventing and Treating Chronic Disease (Brussels, September 15–18, 1996).

Sharpe, Rochelle. "FDA Clarifies Rules on Drugs, Supplements." *Wall Street Journal* (April 27, 1998).

Tyler, Varro. *The New Honest Herbal* (Philadelphia: George Stickley, 1988).

Index